Do
Your
Om
Thing

Do Your Om Thing

*Bending Yoga Tradition
to Fit Your Modern Life*

Rebecca Pacheco

HARPER WAVE

An Imprint of HarperCollins*Publishers*

This book is written as a source of information only. The information contained in this book should by no means be considered a substitute for the advice of a qualified medical professional, who should always be consulted before beginning any new diet, exercise, or other health program. All efforts have been made to ensure the accuracy of the information contained in this book as of the date published. The author and the publisher expressly disclaim responsibility for any adverse effects arising from the use or application of the information contained herein.

HarperCollins books may be purchased for educational, business, or sales promotional use. For information, please e-mail the Special Markets Department at SPsales@harpercollins.com.

FIRST EDITION

Designed by Leah Carlson-Stanisic

Library of Congress Cataloging-in-Publication Data

Pacheco, Rebecca.
    Do your om thing : bending yoga tradition to fit your modern life / Rebecca Pacheco.
        pages   cm
    Includes bibliographical references.
    1. Yoga.   2. Spirituality.   3. Spiritual life.   4. Well-being.   I. Title.
    BL1238.52.P33   2015
    181'.45—dc23   2014044390

ISBN: 978-0-06-227337-6

15 16 17 18 19   OV/RRD   10 9 8 7 6 5 4 3 2 1

For my Vavó

Contents

Part Four: The Spirit

Introduction

This is the part where I tell you that yoga will change your life. Where I enumerate all the ways in which the yoga path will make you happier, healthier, and calmer. I'll use words like *bliss* and *abundance* to describe your newfound or rejuvenated yoga self, which you will visualize as glowing, ethereal, and, of course, fit and sexy. I will suggest that I embody all of these qualities and more.

As a practicing yogi for more than half my lifetime, surely I possess mystical characteristics to elevate me above the realms of reality, and once I dedicated myself to the sacred art of yoga (by this, we mostly assume I am referring to impressive-looking stretches), I never again got stressed or sick. (Sickness is so uninspiring, you know.) Never has someone I loved with every piece of my heart chakra dumped me on my ass. And I certainly never worry about trivial things like parking tickets or calories. I shun entire food groups and think you should, too. In fact, I believe there is a direct correlation between levels of enlightenment attained by a yogi and amount of food groups eschewed. I smile incessantly—from the hour I awake to the blissful (there's that word again) moments before nodding off into a deep sleep, where I am visited in my dreams by auspicious signs, auras, and gurus—possibly even Deepak Chopra.

There's just one problem: I think the word *bliss* is woefully overused in yoga circles. And everyone knows that if you want Deepak Chopra to show up in a dream, you need to book him at least two years in advance. So, I guess that's two problems, really.

There's also the predicament that what I've described isn't actually yoga; it's bullshit. Moreover, even if the imagined yoga utopia were true, it wouldn't really help us understand the core of *what* yoga is and *why* it's useful anywhere off a yoga mat, which is where most of our lives are lived. What about yoga practice leads to physical, mental, and spiritual transformation in real life?

As you may have noticed, the title of this book is *Do Your Om Thing*; this should not be confused with *Do What I Tell You to Do*. There are plenty of yoga books of the Do-What-I-Tell-You-to-Do variety, especially today, in the era of modern yoga when new styles and interpretations emerge all the time. This year's Vinyasa was last year's Power Yoga. Before that, Bikram was all the rage, which previously unseated Ashtanga. Many of these books, new and old, serve as remarkable resources, and you can find my favorites in the Recommended Resources section. This just isn't that type of book.

This book (or, its author) understands that you will occasionally get stressed out, overscheduled, come down with the flu, or possibly dumped on your ass by someone you love with every piece of your heart chakra. Swaddling yourself in lululemon and standing on your head will not change this. Believe me, I've tried. It might make you feel better for a short period, but it won't change your life—nor will becoming vegan, losing ten pounds, going gluten free, or giving up your corporate job. Please don't interpret this as bad news. It's excellent news! It's the liberating reality by which you can finally merge your real life and yoga life. Because the only thing that can bring you the type of enduring peace and balance that ancient yogis sought, called *samadhi* or enlightenment, is the authentic state of you being *you*. Dr. Suess said it perfectly, "Today you are you, that is truer than true. There is no one alive who is Youer than You!"

You are a human being, meaning you are flawed, prone to illness and aging, and inclined to wake up some days and want to pull the covers over your head until this whole thing called life blows over. Adjustments to your outer life, such as diet, wardrobe, and salary, won't change this much for a sustained period. Of course, we should strive to eat healthfully (more on this later), take pride in our appearance, and feel our work is valued fairly, but the intention behind our choices and the relationship we have with ourselves, independent of body weight, fashion sense, or job title, is more important, both to the practice of yoga and to your overall happiness. In other words, your inner life, the one with which yoga is chiefly concerned, changes your experience of everything. The fundamental problem for modern yogis is how to understand the ways in which yoga influences our inner life at a time when yoga's largest and most popular appeals are to our exterior: our bodies, clothes, juice cleanses, and physical poses.

I don't want to diminish the importance of a fulfilling and healthy external life through yoga practice or a healthy lifestyle. Good physical health and confidence are essential to greater well-being and mind/body balance. I love how yoga supports and cultivates these qualities. I'm an athlete, often happiest when challenging my physical limits. As a teacher, I am known for pushing my students' boundaries both physically and mentally. I regularly coach athletes, including professionals and Olympians, helping them use yoga to gain an edge in competition. I also answer the calls of new moms who know yoga can help them get their bodies back after childbirth, along with people who seek other physical improvements, such as core strength, flexibility, less back pain. You name it.

But these goals represent only a fraction of what yoga has to offer. The fittest athletes and most seasoned yogis I know will concur that their lives and performances are most elevated by the states of mental and spiritual clarity evoked by yoga, as opposed to physical performance. Yoga is not about performance. It's about practice, on your mat *and* in your life. If you want to get better at anything, what should you do? Practice. Confidence, compassion, awareness, and joy—if you want more of these—and who doesn't?—yoga offers the skills to practice them. Not to mention have you ever heard someone say, "OMG, my life is so much better now that I can do Astavakrasana!" I didn't think so. Yoga is about attaining a clearer sense of who you are, how you feel, what you want, and how you interact with the world around you. It does enlighten and brighten your whole life, but only if it comes from you, from the inside out—not from a yoga teacher or guru pedaling their agenda on you.

Maybe you have a corporate job, croissant habit, or religious faith that doesn't condone worshipping Ganesha (the playful elephant-headed deity found in many yoga studios). Somewhere along your yogic path, you intuited that you should feel guilty about these perceived inconsistencies with your yoga practice. You developed a hunch that "real yogis" don't wear suits or eat meat. They never have fat days or episodes of Facebook stalking an ex. They don't drink too much wine or lie awake at night worried about bills. You might think this, but you would be wrong.

These assumptions are part of our collective perception of modern yoga, which often only serve to broaden the chasm between who we are in yoga class and who we are outside of it. But at yoga's core, it seeks to *connect us to life* in a compassionate way—not ignore swaths of it that don't fit an idealized image. I don't believe in imposing or preaching a blanket approach to everyone to keep some kind of yoga scorecard. It's important that we have opportunities to consider, understand, and question our assumptions about yoga and how it informs the way we live on a daily basis.

To date, modern yoga hasn't successfully resolved how it aligns with the demands of real life, nor should it. This isn't yoga's job; it's ours. We are the stewards of modern yoga, and we need to pay attention to where it's going. Unfortunately, reading a tome of yoga philosophy—which originated several millennia ago—isn't as exciting as a hot yoga class. Meanwhile, modern yoga philosophy, which can fuse everything from New Age principles to Christianity to Native American healing rituals to psychology, can be more perplexing. These updated approaches to yoga philosophy are the creations of one teacher who found a combination of ideologies inspiring, but that doesn't mean they are universally inspiring. It's not that these new interpretations and styles of yoga are wrong, bad, or "un-yogic"; it's just that they often prioritize the teacher's style or brand of yoga, rather than the honest path of the student.

This book explores the ancient study of yoga from the only perspective that really matters: *yours*. You're a modern yogi. You have vast interests, responsibilities, and goals. You love yoga or like it a lot. Maybe you teach it. You go to classes and practice poses, but you want to know more. You suspect there's a lot more to yoga than supple hamstrings and nice abs, and you're right. To that end, this book helps frame *how* we think about yoga, without telling anyone *what* to think about yoga. It encourages the modern yogi to understand traditional aspects of this ancient practice and apply them to daily life, without becoming a beatific yoga zombie. Too often the misconception persists that the life-affirming nature of yoga eradicates negativity. It doesn't. The nature of life, fraught with its changes, challenges, and suffering, remains. Yoga should not be confused with positive thinking. It's clear thinking.

Through yoga, with its practical set of skills and ethics, perception does change, and major transformation happens. The obstacles and *fluctuations of the mind*—as the yoga sage, Patanjali, called them—hold less sway. Not because a cultlike yoga power brainwashes us to ignore negativity, but because our steadfast brain and attuned body learn to make better choices—about everything—from where we direct our concentration, to what we eat, to how we work, to whom we love. Mastery of the mind is the purpose of yoga, and its most basic description is defined as just that, as being a *science of the mind*. The first step to practicing yoga authentically is to acknowledge that you are not perfect. You live in your life, and you are you. Rather than a limitation or letdown, this is a relief and a privilege.

This book is comprised of four sections: (1) An accessible background on yoga philosophy; (2) a section related to the body as yoga tradition views it, made of five layers, or *koshas*, and seven *chakras*, and how to balance and integrate each of these; (3) a section on the mind, which shares realistic meditation advice for the modern, multitasking human (that's you); and, finally, (4) a section explaining yoga's spiritual roots and the profound impact they can have on day-to-day life, by serving as a spiritual anchor of their own or strengthening and supporting a personal faith or spiritual practice you already have. Because in the end, this is what we're really looking for—a connection to our spirits that's full of light, freedom, and inspiration.

Along the way, we'll also get tips and insight from some amazing yogis and experts, and I will offer you my own pointers and questions to help you reflect on your journey. Above all, my goal for you is to understand that yoga doesn't require you to seek anything you don't already possess. Remember that everything you need is exactly where you are, in this moment, holding this book. (Thank you, from the bottom of my heart, by the way, for picking up this book.)

The word *yoga* originates from the Sanskrit verb *yuj* meaning to yoke, unite, or join together. This synergy of your real life and yoga life, inner and outer worlds, true Self with the collective consciousness, is the path to enlightenment, the purpose of yoga, and the beautiful experience of doing *your* om thing.

Part One

Yoga:
Ancient and Modern

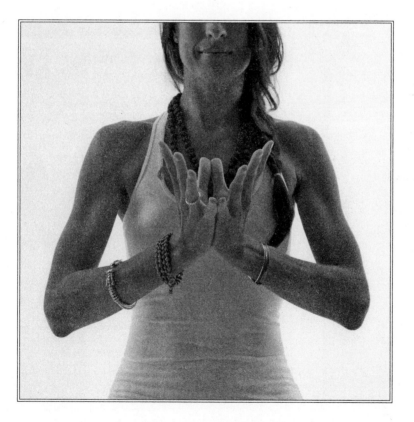

CHAPTER 1

The Making of a Modern Yogi

I began writing this book at the age of sixteen, which is not to say I was some kind of teen prodigy but, rather, a slightly eccentric kid who took up yoga early, then watched closely as it grew into a cultural phenomenon, providing the backdrop for much of my life and fodder for this book.

I attended my first class in the mid-1990s, a lone teenager tucked into a kindly cadre of white-haired retirees on Cape Cod, in Massachusetts. I still wonder how I must have looked to them, young enough to be their granddaughter, attending a weekly yoga class at the local recreation center, where I played indoor youth soccer a few years earlier. I was the only girl on my team back then, and the boys were all smaller and quicker than me. They never passed the ball. To make matters worse, the sleeves of my jersey were too short for my gangly arms, so I was bigger and slower, with a jersey to accentuate this fact. *Great.* Despite being a natural athlete later on, those Saturday afternoons of memory are marked by feeling like a clumsy orangutan in a pack of sporty gazelles in Umbro shorts. (I digress). My point is that yoga was not cool or stylish or popular. And I loved it anyway. Possibly, this is *why* I loved yoga. It seemed like a closely kept, exotic secret.

Today, the secret is out. Yoga's ascendance in popularity outside its birthplace in India began in earnest with the flower children of the 1960s and grew during subsequent decades. In the '90s, when I discovered it, yoga was more visible and available, but it remained a mostly alternative pursuit, for New Age types, former hippies, and aspirant hippies. Even the concept of a studio dedicated exclusively to the practice of yoga wouldn't exist in most cities for several years to come. Until then, yoga was largely found in recreation centers, community halls, church basements, and a growing number of health clubs. (This not-too-distant era also predated specialized yoga mats, stylish pants, snug-fitting tops, and nonskid, toeless socks.) The paparazzi hadn't yet begun to stalk yoga studios in New York and L.A. to snap photos of celebrities with sunglasses in place, mat nonchalantly slung over a shoulder, a look that a popular yoga blogger has coined PDY: Public Displays of Yoga. The sheer fact that I can write a sentence including *yoga*, *paparazzi*, and *popular yoga blogger* is evidence of a dramatic shift in the zeitgeist. When I discovered yoga in a community center at the age of sixteen, there were no celebrities practicing yoga (that I knew of). But this was all about to change. By 1998, the cultural barometer of music, fashion, and fitness trends, Madonna, pledged to maintain her chiseled physique exclusively through yoga and subsequently feng shuied a vast collection of cardio equipment out of her home. The material girl had gone spiritual. In 2001, another very recognizable face graced the cover of the most recognizable magazine in the world: supermodel Christy Turlington on the cover of *Time*, with a headline hailing the "exercise cum meditation trend" that was sweeping the nation. Yet, even with celebrities publicly lauding yoga's benefits around the corner, no one could have predicted the incarnation of "yoga celebrities." Our role models were

B.K.S. Iyengar and Pattabhi Jois, two forefathers of modern yoga. Both were trained by a man named Krishnamacharya and usually photographed in remote areas of southern India wearing loincloths or bloomers.

As for me, I would have been less out of place in that community center if one or more of the following things were true of my first yoga class: (1) I wasn't a teenager. (2) I wasn't sitting on a beach towel in lieu of a yoga mat. (In my defense, the flyer advertising the class recommended a beach towel if you didn't own a proper mat—not that this helped my situation.) (3) I was accompanied by a bohemian parent who practiced yoga, made granola, and wore Birkenstocks. This may come as a surprise, but I don't have a parent like this. My mom maintains an impressive vegetable garden, but she finds tofu offensive, cannot bear the sight of clog shoes of any kind, and has yet to do yoga. My dad is a classically trained chef and career restaurateur. He is not a fan of substituting staple ingredients like butter and eggs for coconut oil or applesauce. These are the nonyogi parents I was allotted, and I love them. (4) I was accompanied by a fellow yoga-curious teenager. This is a ludicrous suggestion for obvious reasons. Teenagers in the '90s talked on the phone for hours, which was plugged into a wall, and made mix tapes for each other. They didn't explore ancient spiritual practices among a gaggle of senior citizens.

I sought my first yoga class for the same reasons any teenager does anything: I was curious, and I knew of someone older and cooler who did it. Jill was the older sister of a friend who embodied cool for me. Initially, I attributed this to the fact that she was in college and possessed a higher social standing through things I lacked, such as a driver's license, shiny blond hair, skinny legs, clear skin, and two separate and well-defined eyebrows. Thankfully, I soon realized these weren't the reasons people beamed when they talked about Jill, and they did beam.

Jill stood apart from the flock. She seemed to care little about how others regarded her legs or anything else, the stuff that consumes a teenager. People brightened around her and talked about the interesting things she did. Even guys sometimes bypassed her blondeness and shininess in favor of the fact that she sang in a rock band or played lacrosse. She didn't look like everyone else, nor did she try. One summer she chopped off all her hair, then wore funky head scarves. When the other college girls started wearing more makeup, Jill wore less. When dainty necklaces from Tiffany adorned their necks, Jill opted for colorful beaded ones made by her friends. She talked about things that excited her, which were not the things that excited other women her age—as best I could gather (while eavesdropping on the older girls at my summer job on the ferryboat where we all worked)—these subjects usually topped out at boys and getting drunk in beach dunes with boys. Jill was beautiful, yes, but her beauty was an afterthought—a parenthetical statement to the stuff that really turned heads—a lightness about her that preceded everything else. Jill understood things I knew I needed to know, like how to care less about what people think; do even the most ordinary things with a hint of a smile, sparkle, or something that says *I am who I am, and I wouldn't have it any other way*; and seek inspiring life experiences—above a din of peer voices. Jill did yoga. I thought there might be a connection between this and the type of person I hoped I'd grow up to be. That's how it started.

Before that first class began, a funny thing happened. The teacher arrived, and she didn't seem to notice how bizarre I looked—the kid on a beach towel, mentally playing back the soccer highlight reel, recalling every clumsy move. Carol was petite and sprightly, with salt-and-pepper hair shorn close in the fashion of a Buddhist nun. Her skin appeared lit from within and creased with expertly placed wrinkles. She looked at me—possibly *through* me—with an expression that was both penetratingly serious and reassuringly gentle.

This kid needs to be here, she said. Not aloud. But, I swear I heard it. And, that was that. At the behest of no one, I'd found yoga, and despite all the reasons to feel out of place because of the uncertain adolescent swirl that follows any adolescent everywhere, I felt perfectly at home. To say this class changed my life would be an unbearably hokey yoga cliché, which I cannot bring myself to utter even if it's true. (OK, it's true.) The changes weren't immediate or dramatic. Yet, when I look back, they were there. In some ways, contemporary yoga and I grew up together. We went through some awkward stages and some graceful ones. We were curious, spiritual, and earnest and—though embarrassing to admit—obsessive, sanctimonious, and hypocritical at times.

I continued my practice and study of yoga during the rest of high school, attending classes when I could. (It was easier when I was back home on Cape Cod, from boarding school in Connecticut, and once I had a license.) I recall justifying the cost of class as a forgone movie ticket because that's what I would have bought with my entertainment dollars instead, and the two were about the same price. I used the bookstore gift certificates I received at Christmas for yoga books and eventually swapped my magazine subscription from *Seventeen* to *Yoga Journal*. I acquainted myself with the serious yogis inside, often pictured in white turbans or black Speedos or both.

In college, I discovered Ashtanga, a vigorous and disciplined style of yoga, which made me a more committed and acrobatic yogi on the mat and arguably less fun of a person off it. Some college students take work-study in the library too seriously (don't even try to sneak in a snack or flirt with your bio lab partner on the Quiet Floor). For me, it was yoga. I equated seriousness with sincerity, and I applied myself to yoga as I did to most things, like academics and sports, where I was focused and intolerant of failure. In this regard, Ashtanga and I were a perfect fit. I liked its meticulous progression through one series of demanding poses to the next series of more-demanding poses. It was regimented and clear, and I found this liberating, especially once everyone in the room knew the sequences. Then, we could breathe and move together, feeling connected without social niceties or actual conversation. I liked the feeling of a bond that didn't require knowing anyone's hometown or sharing a hallway bathroom. Yoga was my own thing in college, if for no other reason than the fact that my peers weren't doing it.

Meanwhile, the classes I took in yoga philosophy and Eastern religions suggested that what I did on my mat paled in comparison to how I lived off it. Yoga was not a sport or form of fitness, and it was gauche to suggest it was. I didn't dare call it a workout. No one did back then. As best as I could gather, I should have dedicated myself to the mastery of my body into impressive pretzel shapes, but once I got there, I was supposed to feel utterly unaffected by said mastery. The poses were not the point, I knew. Yet, the true point escaped me.

I wasn't sure where to go for clarification. My yoga teachers weren't talking about the ancient philosophic roots of yoga that I studied in my college courses, and my philosophy professors sure as heck weren't talking about the pretzel yoga I learned in Ashtanga class. These two yogas: old and the new, inner and outer, mostly spiritual and mostly physical were surely related yet markedly different.

I grappled with the contrast between my real life and my yoga life: from what I ate, to what I believed (or didn't) about God, how I dressed, to how I handled negative emotions I assumed were unyogic. I tried to speak more softly, at times affecting an embarrassingly peaceful lilt like my yoga teachers. In case you missed it, yoga teachers during this early yoga boom often affected weird accents, an imperceptible dialect that sounded a little like a fortune-teller reading Shakespeare while stoned. I felt guilty when I strayed from a strictly vegetarian diet. I worried about drinking alcohol. (Did being in college give me a pass?) My inherited family car was a gas-guzzling SUV. I was harming the environment, and this was obviously bad karma. Should I give up driving altogether? How would I get to my summer job?

My questions about a career path and listening to gangster rap only confused me more. Were Tupac and Biggie putting me at odds with becoming the yogi I wanted to be? Have you listened to the lyrics that fueled the infamous East Coast/West Coast feud of this era? Great for rap. Bad for *ahimsa*, the yoga teaching of non-violence. Were designer clothes and makeup lowly distractions from the spiritual path? *Who* says all this exactly?

I briefly visited India my junior year of college, and gained a new perspective on my practice. I was in the south of the country, just a few towns away from the birthplace of Ashtanga yoga, yet no one seemed interested in intricate balances, binds, or knotted poses, just sitting and breathing. Once, we chanted on a beach at sunrise. When I asked the guru what we were chanting, he wouldn't say.

Shortly thereafter I began teaching my peers, and soon, classes grew to include more than one hundred students, staff, and faculty on our study abroad program. In the years to follow, I graduated from college, moved to Boston, and worked a nine-to-five job by day and became a properly certified yoga teacher by night. I became the youngest master-level teacher at one of the most famous yoga studios in the world, and I worked closely with some of the biggest names in modern yoga. I learned a lot, and I saw a lot. Of both yoga's best and its most hypocritical. Sometimes, I became disheartened by the way some use yoga as another medium for posturing and puffery. But, always, I returned to its power to impart health and meaning on the mat and in modern life for anyone seeking either.

I return to what I have learned repeatedly and empirically on my journey: Yoga improves and enriches lives. When practiced in earnest, yoga can synthesize every aspect of who we are and how we interact with the world, leading to a more authentic, compassionate, and joyful experience. A karmic yogi who truly lived his practice, Mahatma Gandhi, put it this way: "Happiness is when what you think, what you do, and what you say are in harmony."

You know the physical benefits of yoga already, so I won't belabor them too much. They are the primary factors for most people to start doing yoga. They include but are not limited to improved flexibility, stress reduction, weight loss/management, more energy, sounder sleep, and the rehabilitation of injuries or imbalances in the body. Back pain is the most common.

My athlete clients comment that they experience fewer injuries, improved focus, and enhanced performance with yoga. Meanwhile a venture capitalist student of mine, who's a father of three, once reported with satisfaction that soon after investing in our regular yoga sessions, he could twist around enough in the driver's seat of his car to see all three kids sitting behind him. Before yoga, he could turn only far enough to see two. Then, one day, there was his littlest, smiling brightly. Now, he could see her. People generally feel better when they do yoga of any kind, in any capacity. It strengthens bodies and minds, and it's like weight lifting for the spirit. Yogis twist more easily, but even better, they see more clearly the beauty around them or sitting in the backseat.

But practicing yoga for its myriad health benefits, while wonderful, is limiting. It's akin to traveling to Italy, with all its exquisitely fresh, local cuisine, to eat PB&J sandwiches the whole time. You might enjoy the sights, capture breathtaking photos, and take in iconic art and architecture with your own eyes, but you wouldn't taste Italy. You'd miss luscious tomatoes, aromatic basil, and rich olive oil. You'd forgo recipes perfected over generations and relinquish plates of pasta, pizza, or *zuppa* created with love. You'd depart with a sinking suspicion you were missing something. You'd feel unsatisfied. Still a little hungry. Because to experience Italy is to eat there, much like doing yoga is to nourish the spirit, not just the body.

The emphasis on yoga's physical practice belies its most fundamental intention—the one from which we can benefit most—an ability to slow down our overstimulated, overtired, incessantly multitasking minds. Internal quiet and connection to our deepest self form the essence of yoga. It's not fancy. It doesn't balance on one arm. But it's the plain truth of yoga's purpose, and *it will change your life.*

Originally written in Sanskrit as *chitta vritti nirodhah*, the purpose of yoga is "to still the fluctuations of the mind," per *The Yoga Sutras of Patanjali*, a foundational yoga text written roughly 2,000 years ago. Everything else, such as the flexibility and fitness, is secondary.

This is the crux of the modern yogi's dilemma: We sense that yoga is more than the physical postures, yet we rarely see evidence of this. Instead, portrayals of yoga disproportionately favor physical images, often conveyed by beautiful, bendy, waifish model types, in impressively contorted poses. And while I may serve as that bendy model at times, I can assure you, no amount of makeup, Photoshop, or chicken cutlets stuffed into my sports bra ever make me feel whole, authentic, or happy.

How can I attempt to personalize for you an exercise cum meditation trend embraced and idealized by pop culture? First, we must agree on what yoga is. We know it's a state of connection with the purpose of calming the mind, but how do we get there—to that peaceful, uncluttered, awakened state where the self-judgment, multitasking, and status seeking cease? It's not a certain type of yoga or pose that will get us there. It's not achieved by blindly following a guru or changing your diet. It's the cultivation of an inner life that feels whole. Yoga doesn't manufacture a feeling of completeness; it offers tools for becoming present enough to realize it's been there all along. So let's search beyond what we see most of yoga and explore what we need most *in our lives*. The tools in these pages are now yours, too. When they are put to use, they help us better understand yoga and experience its benefits beyond the mat, through the fullness of life.

CHAPTER 2

The Eight Limbs:
Walking an Ancient Path in Modern Life

It's virtually impossible to distill thousands of years of yoga phi-losophy down to a few pages, but I'm going to do my best. And I'm going to try to make it fun! Let's start with the understanding that yoga is meaningful beyond its poses, which we've established is true. Above all, because we *feel* it, whether we've been doing yoga for a few days or several decades. This intuition is the reason you picked up this book. The pivotal question to ask now is: how is yoga meaning-ful beyond its poses? How can we practice yoga beyond the physical experience? How can we pick up where a typical yoga class leaves off? In other words, what do we need to know to get the most out of our yoga and, by extension, our lives?

The best way to answer these questions is to refer to some of yoga's deepest roots, and then bend an ancient tradition filled with wisdom and pragmatism to fit our modern lives. If you've been practicing yoga for a while, gone on a retreat, attended teacher training, or have taught yoga, you may already be familiar with the aforementioned *Yoga Sutras*, a collection of aphorisms or little threads of advice (*sutra* means thread in Sanskrit) that outline the key tenets of yoga. If not, here's a quick review.

The Indian scholar Patanjali is credited with compiling the *Yoga Sutras* around 400 CE. Patanjali didn't invent yoga; rather, he transcribed an oral tradition already in existence into one cohesive text. It's like an instruction manual, albeit a rich and illuminating one. In it, Patanjali specifically outlines the eight-limbed yoga path, which guides yogis toward inner and outer peace through a series of simple practices and directions. It's a map, leading us toward a life of meaning and contentment, using all facets of yoga, not just the bendy ones we see on Instagram. The eight-limbed path includes the following practices:

Yamas: attitudes toward the world
Niyamas: attitudes toward self
Asanas: yoga postures
Pranayama: breathwork
Pratyhara: withdrawal of the senses or turning inward
Dharana: concentration
Dhyana: meditation
Samadhi: enlightenment

While these concepts may have originated long ago, their benefits are no less relevant and accessible today. We intuitively understand that having a personal code of ethics and set of healthy behaviors gives us dignity and inner peace. Alternatively, we understand the dangers of losing connection to our internal compass of integrity of soul. When we practice any one of the limbs, we honor the tradition of yoga and connect more deeply and readily to our best selves.

Nevertheless, the *Sutras* isn't exactly a page-turning read, and anybody who tells you otherwise is bluffing. The sutras are essential, educational, and insightful, but they are not a rollicking good time. Thus, I present to you my take on the eight limbs of yoga with a touch of rollick and special attention to how they might be applicable to your life today.

Limb 1: Yamas | Attitudes Toward the World

Modern yogis are often surprised to learn that the first priority of the eight-limbed yoga path isn't physical and has nothing to do with touching one's toes. In fact, the asanas, the postures we're most accustomed to doing and seeing, don't show up until third on the list.

The first stage or limb focuses on how we treat others and relate to the world. It's about ethics. The yamas teach compassion for everyone and everything around us, and they have little to do with what happens on the yoga mat (which makes sense when you consider that yoga mats didn't exist 2,500 years ago). As with many Sanskrit words, the translation of *yamas* varies, but "attitudes toward the world" is an accurate and encompassing one, so let's use it. The following ethical teachings make up the yamas: *ahimsa* (non-harming), *satya* (truthfulness), *asteya* (non-stealing), *brahmacharya* (abstinence), and *aparigraha* (greedlessness).

At first glance, these guidelines would appear to be self-explanatory. But let's explore these lessons a little deeper and look at how they translate into our modern yoga practice, beyond literal translations and traditional interpretations. After all, you may not be interested in becoming celibate. Just a hunch.

Ahimsa: Non-Harming
Upon graduating from medical school, new doctors take the Hippocratic oath, which is a pledge to practice medicine ethically. Its central purpose is widely understood to be: *first do no harm*. In some ceremonies, candidates from different countries recite a portion of

the oath in their native languages. It's a jubilant occasion, the culmination of years of painstaking work, sacrifice, and sleep deprivation
in the name of healing others. The gravity of becoming a doctor is
more momentous than that of becoming a yogi, but the first priority
is the same. Do no harm. There's no formal oath for us, but implicit
in the practice of yoga is the understanding that we minimize harm
to others and ourselves whenever possible. This is called ahimsa.

Ahimsa, meaning non-harming or non-violence, reminds us not
to act violently, speak carelessly or maliciously, or think harmful
thoughts. *Non-violence* is the common translation; however, *non-
harming* is a more effective and inclusive definition. *Harm* encapsu-
lates more, which is not to say that modern yogis need more rules,
but we do need greater opportunities to practice mindful living.

Ahimsa is yoga's primary practice: the first ethical guideline of
the first limb. It makes clear the idea that yoga means nothing unless
it creates peace for you and others in the world. "Practice should not
be separated from living and living at all times should be one's practice," the Zen master Sheng Yen once said.

The eight limbs are precepts, as opposed to rules or commandments, yet they bear a striking resemblance to both. Through them,
the yogi sees and interacts with the world in a thoughtful and compassionate way. It goes without saying that yogis shouldn't commit
acts of violence. (Let's just make a blanket statement that people
shouldn't commit acts of violence?) Yet, avowed non-violent people
harm each other all the time, in subtle and insidious ways. Ahimsa
teaches us to consider the impact of our actions, words, and intentions through a lens of self-awareness, reflection, and compassion.

Imagine how much more peaceful living would be if your mind
was free of toxic thoughts. Road rage, gossip, or glancing in the mirror and saying unthinkably cruel things to the reflection staring
back at you are all subtly harmful behaviors that erode our sense of
peace in daily life. Actions like these pale in comparison to physical
violence, but each one plants a seed of harm that over time sprouts

more negative feelings and thought patterns (known as *samskaras*). This isn't to say that having a fat day means you're a yoga fraud. It happens. But before we even start to talk about touching our toes or standing on our hands, the *Sutras* advises us to break unhealthy mental patterns and construct new ones. If you wanted to distill the yoga path into a single, rudimentary piece of advice (or if you suspect this book might be crap and you want the one-sentence takeaway), this is it: Ahimsa *is the most important aspect of yoga*. Cause less harm; cultivate more compassion. Your life and yoga will thank you.

The practice of non-harming represents the first stage of becoming more enlightened. It benefits every aspect of our being: physical, energetic, emotional, intellectual, and spiritual. It enhances any environment: home, work, school, and local and global communities. And it's the yoga equivalent of the Golden Rule, with opportunities to practice it everywhere. It may not relate to physical flexibility, but it has everything to do mental and emotional flexibility—with ourselves, our neighbors, and the world.

As modern yogis, we're often led to believe that nonviolence takes specific, predetermined forms, causing us to wrestle with questions of personal ethics. Politically, for instance, we might assume we should oppose abortion, capital punishment, or war. Meanwhile, in a yoga environment, yoga teachers, studios, and resources often cite ahimsa as the primary argument in support of veganism, thereby avoiding the killing of animals for food, clothing, cosmetics, and more. While all these compassionate positions are admirable, drawing a hard line for all yogis in all situations and all geographic locations (regardless of climate or socioeconomic factors) overlooks the importance of each individual's journey. We each walk our own path and, by elevating our consciousness along the way, come to the best conclusions for the lives we lead. Through self-reflection and by applying an ahimsa-inspired outlook to all areas of life, we can choose how best to grocery shop, vote, eat, or make any other decision. I happen to be pro-choice and opposed to the death penalty. I arrived at these beliefs by determining what I believe will cause the least amount of suffering. All we can control is our own corner of the universe. Ourselves. The goal is to create peace in our little corner. And remember, the sutras are guiding principles rather than rules with black or white distinctions. Because life is rarely black or white, and the yogi is better served learning about him- or herself and making choices that align with the rest of his or her life rather than abiding by rules set by others.

I mentioned that the urge to protect all living creatures becomes so strong in many yogis that they simply cannot bear to eat animals. This is an honorable choice and beneficial to the environment, but it's not essential that you make the same choice on your yogic journey. You can eat a burger and still practice a mindful lifestyle. There are no spiritual scorecards on the path to enlightenment. The eight limbs are meant to wake us up to our highest good and truest self, which must come from our own personal experience.

Yoga and Buddhism are not the same, but they do share some of the same values and practices. Ahimsa is one of these. Which might make you surprised to learn that His Holiness the Dalai Lama, the spiritual leader of Tibet and the most famous, highest-ranking Buddhist monk in the world (many people view him as an incarnation of the Buddha himself), is neither vegan nor vegetarian. Yet I think few people would suggest that his diet makes him a less compassionate person or a bad example for others when he has dedicated the majority of his life to eliminating suffering for others and teaching compassion around the world. His choice is mindful and connected to all other aspects of his well-being and those of his people, who would likely starve or suffer greatly without eating meat, which is more readily available in Tibet's harsh, isolated climate than year-round vegetables. Each of us lives a cumulative, interdependent life, and as yogis, we must focus on the collective impact of all our actions—large and small. This is what we mean when we say yoga evokes *wholeness*.

Honoring the first yoga priority is simple: be kind. Cause less harm. Create more compassion. You don't have to agree with everyone all the time, but you do need to show respect and expect to receive it in return. Don't be phony or saccharine, but choose your best expressions of kindness toward everyone, as often as possible, each day. Advance this principle by testing yourself to see if you can view more people and situations with eyes of compassion, and not just at the yoga studio or in other environments where everyone is safe, well-behaved, and familiar. The goal is to eventually include *all* beings in your compassion. Practice your non-harming attitude when you are exhausted, cranky, and downtrodden, toward people who annoy you. Let the modern yoga world remain seduced by acrobatic yoga poses, while you elevate your consciousness in traffic jams, heated political debates, or the dressing room with that vicious fluorescent lighting and fun house mirror. Practice this yama just as you would an inversion, like a headstand. If you find it challenging, don't give up. Don't judge yourself too harshly. Just start over and keep practicing. When others falter on their path, try your best to show compassion for them and their mistakes.

Finally, it's important not to confuse compassion with martyrdom or a lack of conviction. While we should aim to minimize any amount of harm we bring to the world, we shouldn't attempt to dodge controversy altogether or subject ourselves to the harmful behaviors of others in the name of a higher ideal. That wouldn't be an honest or productive way to live. Yoga wants you to live a safe and dignified life. There's an old ahimsa parable I love, which illustrates this point beautifully:

> *There was once a poisonous snake that terrorized a tiny village. He bit everyone and everything without discretion: women, children, and even cherished family pets. One day, a monk visited the village and observed the snake's behavior. Like any good monk, he com-*

mitted to teaching the snake the principle of ahimsa, a core tenet of yogic philosophy (as well as other philosophies and religions of the East). As luck would have it, the snake had a penchant for self-improvement and thoroughly absorbed the monk's teachings. He loved the concept of ahimsa and accepted it wholeheartedly.

The snake stopped biting the villagers cold turkey. It was a big moment of personal evolution for him—but, of course, there was a downside. The villagers, fueled by years of abuse and fear, now exploited the snake's personal truce and practice of ahimsa. They threw rocks at him. They poked him with sticks. They generally made his life miserable. One year later, the monk returned to find the snake bruised, beaten, and starving.

"What happened to you!" exclaimed the gentle teacher. It pained him to see his former student in such a predicament. The predator had, indeed and unfortunately, become the prey, as the adage goes. Sad and slightly exasperated, the snake replied, "You taught me the principle of non-violence. YOU taught me not to bite people!"

The snake had a point. The monk taught him to harm no living thing and show unconditional care and compassion at all times. Under no circumstances was he to create more hostility and violence in a world so fraught with both already. How could the monk respond? The snake was a good and noble student.

"Ahhh, my son, I did teach you not to bite people," the monk conceded.

Then, he lowered his voice to indicate the sharing of an important secret, "But I never said you couldn't hissssss."

DO YOUR OM THING: PRACTICE KINDNESS

- In what ways do my thoughts, words, and actions cause harm (e.g., at home, work, school, to myself and others)?
- What's one negative thought pattern (samskara) that I need to change to create more peace in my life and the world?
- Instead of being a martyr/victim, how can I respectfully hiss to protect myself?

Satya: Truthfulness

Gloria Steinem famously said, "The truth will set you free, but first it will piss you off." Maybe you can relate. Sometimes, truth hits hard and fast, knocking the wind out of you. The air vacates your lungs, and you wonder how a ruthless linebacker snuck up on you without warning. The truth also surfaces gradually, setting up quiet residence in an overlooked corner of your heart, patiently waiting for attention. Truth will sit for days, months, or years, until the moment you acknowledge her presence. *Hi. I'm over here. I've been waiting for you to notice me.* Living the life of the yogi implies that we act from this moment of awareness. Once we know truth (satya), we must live it. Avoiding or ignoring the truth creates discord in the hearts and lives of ourselves and others.

The obvious interpretation of satya is: don't lie. Like "don't be violent," "don't lie" is pretty much standard operating procedure for being a decent human being. Most of us have been taught not to lie from a very young age. We know that lying leads to trouble, weakens relationships, and generally makes us feel anxious. But not telling lies is just one aspect of this yama. It also applies to conveying a lack of truthfulness through words unsaid, commonly known as lies of omission. It dissuades us from gossip and other forms of communication containing a lack of truth or integrity. And, in a broader context, satya is about learning our own essential truths, the inarguable, the beautiful, and not beautiful pieces of self that exist whether we like it or not. Our personal truths can't be construed or convoluted (try as we might when they are painful or inconvenient), and their reality is so simple and enduring that when we think about them or utter them aloud, every cell in our body perks up to listen. *Here, here,* they say. It could be our true calling, true love, or the truest piece of advice we've ever heard and will never forget. We know truth when we hear it. We nod. No further explanation needed. *YES*, we think. *That's it!* Like seeing a painting or piece of clothing and feeling as though it were created especially for you. The truth fits. When you live it, it feels good. When you don't, all those untruths feel itchy, too tight, and ugly. This is not to say that the truth is always comfortable. Not even close. Just refer back to Gloria Steinem's quote. Living from your truth is the most liberating experience in the world, but getting to that point can be a difficult, sometimes painful, process. Lucky for us, we have a truth-seeking, spirit-strengthening, no-b.s.-taking practice called yoga to help.

We come to know our personal truths by way of experience and study: through quotes or scripture, from a teacher or spiritual guide, through art, and, most of all, through the wisdom of our own inner voice. To demonstrate what I mean by finding the essential truths in your own life, let me share one of my own, which inspires and informs the way I live.

On my thirtieth birthday, I attended a lecture given by Deepak Chopra. "You must never, ever, use someone else's map," Chopra told us. He was referring to how we lay plans and set intentions, and his point was one I needed to hear. I recalled moments in my career when a linear path or ladder didn't work for me. I'd diverted on occasions. I'd overlapped. I'd explored multiple careers at once. I'd sampled industries that caught my fancy and wondered about others. Sometimes, I felt like the possibilities were endless. Other times,

I worried I was losing my way. I once lived next door to group of Ivy League guys who all studied engineering together and upon graduation worked in engineering at the same company. They seemed to have it together. I envied them. Their choice was so tidy and simple. Study X, get a job doing Y. Mine was the opposite—too many interests, passions, and possibilities intersecting and leading who knows where? I felt like I was doing something wrong.

What I eventually came to realize was my truth wasn't their truth. My path wasn't their path. I needed to create my own map. The truth of my calling would reveal itself.

The Buddha famously taught his first students a similar lesson:

Do not believe in anything simply because you have heard it. Do not believe in anything simply because it is spoken and rumored by many. Do not believe in anything simply because it is found written in your religious books. Do not believe in anything merely on the authority of your teachers and elders. Do not believe in traditions because they have been handed down for many generations. But after observation and analysis, when you find that anything agrees with reason and is conducive to the good and benefit of one and all, then accept it and live up to it.

With so much competing information in the world, it's as important as ever to use your personal truth as the ultimate compass. Yoga is the training ground. Listen to your heart. Be honest about what you hear. Then, act. If you don't know what to do, keep listening. Never lie—not explicitly or by omission. Most of all, not to yourself. Use what rings true for you, and trust that your map is unfolding just as it should.

....

DO YOUR OM THING: SEEK THE TRUTH

....

- I will identify one personal truth that is essential to me. It reminds me who I am.
- I will identify one lie I will STOP telling myself immediately.
- I will discover one person, activity, or place that helps me connect to my truth.
- I will reflect on how it feels to speak and live my truth.

....

Asteya: Non-Stealing

Like lying, we learn from an early age that stealing is wrong. Yoga tradition refers to the principle of non-stealing as asteya. It's an easy lesson: don't take what isn't yours (unless it's a few of your sweetheart's French fries—obvious exception). Like many yoga lessons, the application of asteya extends beyond a literal translation. Whether we realize it or not, even the most virtuous among us probably steal something on a daily basis. I was curious about the most common forms of theft, so I posed the question to a dedicated group of modern yogis, my OmGal.com readers.

Beyond material possessions or money, which resources do we steal from each other most?

Here's what they said:

- **Time:** Our most precious resource topped the list. Chronic lateness, departing yoga classes and other commitments early, and tying up others with idle chatter exemplify ways in which we steal time from others and ourselves. Everyone is given the same number of hours in a day. It's how we use them that differ.

- **Attention:** Taking credit that isn't ours or upstaging others is a stealth type of thievery. Attention and recognition are forms of currency that can be shared or stolen, just like money and material goods.
- **Work/Effort:** Who hasn't done work for which they weren't compensated fairly, suffered the sting of plagiarism, or watched an original idea lifted and used as if it were the creativity of another?
- **Space:** Western yogis are very cognizant about personal space, especially those who live in cities, travel frequently, or use public transport. Yoga classes can also be crowded, and there's nothing worse than an invasive neighbor who lacks self-awareness or etiquette. Double-parking a mat when others need a space. Stowing more junk in the yoga room than fits in the overhead compartment. Letting a pool of sweat seep dangerously close to nearby mats. These are all examples of yogis taking more than they need.
- **Energy:** We've all experienced people (even yoga people) who sap energy, steal thunder, or suck the wind out of another's sails. It's deflating and exhausting. Think of it as energy theft, or you may have heard it called *energy vampirism*. No Sanskrit translations needed for this one.

....

DO YOUR OM THING: DON'T STEAL

....

- What is one way I steal from others and how I can I stop?
- Which thoughts, behaviors, or people steal/sap my energy?
- Which of my precious resources do I most need to protect?

....

Brahmacharya: Abstinence

Here's what I know about sex: if it wasn't part of personal ethics, it wouldn't be so scandalous, and if it weren't spiritual, we wouldn't be calling God's name so often while we were doing it.

Truth be told, I know a little more than that about sex. We all do, thankfully. What I mean to say is that being a yogi asks that we consider the integrity of our sexual energy. Sometimes it surprises people that sex is considered within the realm of yoga, but it actually makes perfect sense. Individually and culturally, we think about sex a lot. It's a big part of life. The old myth that a man thinks about sex every seven seconds is just that, a myth, but it's still fairly frequent. Researchers estimate that it's a couple times per hour for men and about half as often for women. And no one bats a flirty eyelash anymore when we hear the advertising credo that *sex sells*—sex in advertising has become de rigueur. Sex is ever-present in our music, entertainment, fashion, and media. Put simply, sex occupies a lot of our attention and energy. It also, vitally, creates life, and, therefore, sustains humanity. It's crucially important. The realm of yoga practice that contemplates the role of sex in our ethical and spiritual lives is called brahmacharya, which typically translates to mean abstinence.

Before you panic, rest assured that I'm not suggesting you forego sex in order to become a more enlightened yogi. Even some of the oldest yoga scriptures make a distinction between the necessary celibacy of ascetic yogis or "forest dwellers" versus "householders." The former retreated from society to meditate in caves, practice yoga in solitude, and curb their sexual desires by channeling their mojo toward more pious pursuits. Meanwhile, the latter maintained families, for which sex is paramount. It's tough to procreate without the creative act of sex, right? Nevertheless, modern yogis have a tendency to categorically overlook this teaching, which is fine. Until it's not. Until the latest guru is caught taking advantage of a student. Until an affair rocks your relationship or family. Until you find yourself in a relationship you no longer want to be in. Until a friend's heart is left in shambles by what was supposed to be a harmless "friends with benefits" arrangement. You'll keep your phone on, all hours. You tell her to call you, not him, when she's lonely or hysterical. You build an arsenal of jokes and asides to keep her from prolonging the damage.

Being unclear, irresponsible, or unfulfilled in our sexual needs, desires, and boundaries wreaks havoc on our emotional and even physical well-being. Yoga teaches us to be more aware of how we see and interact with the world, including between the sheets.

It also helps to broaden the way we think about brahmacharya: not just to include sex, intimacy, infidelity, and flirtation, to name the obvious, but also to think about how abstinence might enhance our lives when applied to areas in which it's needed. Nancy Gilgoff, the first American woman to study Ashtanga yoga in India with Pattabhi Jois and one of the practitioners who brought the practice to the U.S. in the '70s, defines brahmacharya as "welling in the supreme being," which suggests having enough self-restraint to know when to expend energy (sexual or otherwise) and when to well it up and save yourself. (Please excuse the virginal pun.) I don't know about you, but I could stand to practice abstinence more often when it comes to certain perfectionist tendencies of mine. And I can say with certainty that my quality of life vastly improves when I abstain from, for example, too much TV, dairy, sugar, draining personal and professional relationships, or a nasty habit of being overly self-critical. These modern riffs on the traditional teaching of brahmacharya might not be what our yogi ancestors envisioned, but I doubt they envisioned much about the pace and evolution of our lifetime. Everything evolves.

It's hard to say how yoga's image evolved from unshaven armpits and Birkenstocks to bendy sexpots doing near-naked (or totally naked) yoga on the Internet, but it happened. As yoga has gone mainstream, it's also gotten sexier. To many, today's trend toward better-dressed, hipper, hotter, sexed-up yoga feels more current, realistic, and fun. To others, it's a travesty. Both sides have valid reasons. In the end, the practice is less about doing it a certain way and more about being conscious of what you're doing and why you're doing it.

I'll be honest; I don't like sexed-up yoga. Yoga can be sexy, and sex can be yogic (i.e., tantric), especially since flexibility, focus on the present, and feeling good in your own skin increases pleasure, but I prefer that yoga and sex mostly sleep in separate rooms. That's my om thing. It doesn't have to be yours.

So, whether we're teaching a yoga class or taking one, running a small business or running for office, in a relationship or playing the field, this lesson reminds us to be responsible and respectful of how we use our sexual energy. Brahmacharya manifests itself differently for each of us. First and most obviously, it suggests not eroding relationships with infidelity, unclear boundaries, or using sex to fill a void in one's life (e.g., boredom, loneliness, or low self-esteem). Then, there are subtler observances, from keeping the intentions of a yoga teacher's hands-on adjustments of students clear and corrective (not creepy or self-serving) to thinking twice about acting on sexual chemistry during a yoga retreat. In other words, it's important to be aware of what kind of sexual energy we invite or emit in the yoga studio and beyond.

Just as we can be sexually promiscuous by engaging in too many indiscriminate affairs, we can be energetically promiscuous by lacking awareness of how our thoughts, words, and actions influence the relationships and bonds we create. Do we choose our romantic partners out of love and respect or something else? Do we honor our close friendships or take some for granted? Are we present in our commitments—whether romantic, platonic, familial, or professional—or do we "get around" without paying much attention to how our energetic output affects the world around us? Committing ourselves to too many people and obligations in which we're not truly invested can be a form of energetic promiscuity, which runs the risk of making us feel used up and discarded afterward. Ana Forrest, the founder of Forrest Yoga and never one for subtlety, refers to this lack of energetic abstinence as "sacrificial whoring." The term is a little strong, but it underscores the fundamental question that this yama poses: do our bonds align with who we want to be? The yoga path asks us to study where and on what we spend our energy (sexual, creative, and otherwise) because this creates our reality. The principle of brahmacharya encourages us to create mindfully.

....

DO YOUR OM THING:
USE CREATIVE AND SEXUAL ENERGY WITH CARE

....

- Are my sexual relationships respectful of others and myself?
- In which areas of my life am I promiscuous with my creative energy?
- I feel sexy when _____.
- I am most creative when _____.

....

Aparigraha: Greedlessness

Greed never ends well. In its best-case scenario where no one eats too much ice cream and gets nauseous, goes to prison for securities fraud, depletes land of its natural resources, or oppresses a group of people in the name of greater wealth or power, it's still a bleak state of being. When greed goes unchecked, we feel discontent, unfulfilled, and insatiably wanting. No matter how much you have, it will never be enough, and that is a tough way to live. It's a state of perpetual suffering: never content and always wanting more or something different than what you have, or desiring that others have less. It makes us feel separate, small, and constantly at odds with perceived scarcity. We resent people who have the things we want. Yoga helps us see these greedy tendencies (we all have them) and return to a state of generosity. This ethical aspect of yoga is called aparigraha or greed-lessness.

OK, I'll go first: I'm borderline obsessed with sunglasses, sneak-ers, and bangle bracelets. I have more of these objects than one set of eyes, feet, or wrists realistically need. I also hog the blankets at night (in my defense, I don't mean to; I'm asleep). I've gotten better at purging books, but it still feels like I'm giving away part of my soul when I pare down a personal library (even books I've never read nor realistically intend to). I should throw out more of my old photos and love letters. I love sea salt too much. I am always eyeing the cookie with the most chocolate chips. And I cringe sometimes when I catch myself forcing a work opportunity I don't want simply because I can't bear saying no and letting someone else have it. *What if I'm missing out and someone else gets all the credit/compensation/fun?* It's a selfish, silly fear, with which I've learned to make friends and let it go, but its shadow still creeps. I'd cop to more salacious tendencies, but I'm also greedy about word counts, so that's all I can spare.

Whether a harmless fascination with something specific and ma-terial, a greedy emotional tendency, or dangerous habit, learning to evaluate and temper our urges helps us know who we are at our core, release the unhealthy holds they have on us, and increase our expe-rience of contentment (santosha), which we'll talk more about soon.

I had been doing yoga for fifteen years before I heard a teacher mention the concept of aparigraha and integrate it into what we were doing on our mats, which is one way to characterize the missing piece of modern yoga in the bigger picture. We overrepresent the poses' fitness pointers and sex appeal and overlook the ethical and spiri-tual side of the practice. Thankfully, not in Patricia Walden's classes. Walden is the most senior Iyengar teacher in the United States, and even if you've never done Iyengar yoga or had a desire to try its slow, precise (sometimes exacting) approach, your practice (or teacher) has been influenced by its founder, B.K.S. Iyengar. Guruji, as his students called him, practiced yoga daily until the age of ninety-five.

In 2014, at the age of ninety-six, he passed away, leaving an indelible mark on the world. Iyengar helped shepherd yoga's expansion to America from his home in Pune, India, decades ago, and his myriad books remain some of the best resources for students and teachers.

One day, Walden was demonstrating a very advanced, deep, backbend to our Level 5 class, hanging off a chair (Iyengar yoga is big on props such as blocks, straps, blankets, and even chairs) in the kind of pose that looks über impressive, tickles the ego, and can therefore cause injury if done recklessly. She hung upside down, like a bat (albeit a graceful blond one with bright skin and a lithe frame belying her more than sixty years), and raised an authoritative finger.

"Don't be greedy now," she clucked, warning us to honor our bodies and curb the ego's tendency to push or fixate on an unattainable or unhealthy goal. Never one to coddle, Walden wasn't telling us to coast. That is *not* her style, but she was telling us to check ourselves before we wreck ourselves.

The class laughed. We knew too well the risk of being yogis who convince ourselves of validation on the other side of balancing on our hands, head, or chin. Leave it to Walden to illustrate with a single, gently delivered admonishment that we merely transfer our greediness from shoes or handbags to yoga poses when we do this. Yoga is the vehicle. You are the driver.

Of course, this yoga practice of greedlessness stands in sharp contrast to the capitalistic nature of the society in which the modern yogi now lives. This yama teaches us to keep desires in check by not seeking to obtain more than we need. This doesn't mean we can't be prosperous. It doesn't mean that wealth is bad. It asks us to consider the undercurrent of our striving and intention behind it. Is our want for more wealth a desire we have to express ourselves more fully, create opportunity, and provide for others, and ourselves, or is it an insatiable attraction to symbols and status?

Aparigraha also relates to the habit of coveting what isn't ours. Envying someone else's possessions or life is a quick path to unhappiness, and we might think of jealousy as a form of spiritual greed. It's also the least effective of human emotions. Whereas other negative emotions like fear or anger can have positive and productive applications—fear can keep us safe and anger can be a healthy catalyst for change, for example—jealousy is a wounded, lame creature that gnaws away at the heart and contributes nothing in return. It's corrosive and crappy for the person who feels it and has no impact on the person to whom it's directed. Whenever you catch yourself feeling the familiar twinge of jealousy, nip it as quickly as possible. When its toxic fumes are fanned, you will find yourself in a fog of greed.

Aparigraha teaches us to be grateful for the opportunities, experiences, and possessions we have. It's okay to take pleasure in providing for yourself and others through material and spiritual wealth, but recognize when you are following the pull of greedy impulses that deplete your soul rather than strengthen it. Whether it's a pair of overpriced shoes, a bottomless bag of chips, that advanced yoga pose for which you're not ready, the status climb for money but empty of purpose. The easiest way to assuage our personal monsters of greed—Buddhists call these urges "hungry ghosts"—is to flex your gratitude and generosity just like your muscles, every day.

....

DO YOUR OM THING:
CHECK GREED. EXPAND GENEROSITY.

....

- What are my greedy tendencies?
- What form of generosity do the people in my life need from me right now?
- In what ways do I show gratitude to those who are generous to me?

....

Limb 2: Niyamas | Attitudes Toward Self

Following the first stage of yoga, yamas, which coach the yogi on how to view and interact with the world, are the *niyamas*. Often translated as *attitudes toward the self*, self-restraints, or forms of self-discipline, these practices encourage us to treat ourselves with respect. They include: *saucha* (cleanliness), *santosha* (contentment), *tapas* (discipline), *svadhyaya* (self-study), and *isvara pranidhana* (surrender to God/having faith).

Saucha: Cleanliness

The belief that cleanliness is important to spiritual development shows up in many faiths and spiritual practices. "Cleanliness is next to godliness," the Bible says. Pilgrims remove their shoes before entering a temple or circumnavigating a holy site in many traditions. In Christianity, Judaism, and Islam, ablutions serve as ritual cleansings. Meanwhile, yogis have saucha, which traditionally refers to keeping the home of our spirit—the body—clean and healthy but can also extend to our environs.

I joke that Iyengar classes are identifiable not only by their meticulous approach to postural alignment but also by the housekeeping of equipment (to the point that it might be considered compulsive yoga cleanliness disorder). Everything has a place and process in an Iyengar studio, from blocks stacked like miniature skyscrapers of foam or wood, to straps coiled tightly like perfect fiddleheads from the garden, to an elaborate system for folding and stowing the ubiquitous Mexican blankets that have become a staple in many yoga studios. Tassels should face the wall, neat folds facing out, else you will be deemed the most slovenly yogi in all the land. I used to envision Iyengar himself, materializing out of thin air, ready to throw down because the tassels were in disarray. This was just my imagination, of course. But we all know the feelings of disarray that come with a messy house or period of detouring from a clean diet and lifestyle into overindulgence or outright junk.

In Swami Visnu Devananda's *The Complete Illustrated Book of Yoga*, he explains the importance of saucha as it relates to the rest of yoga. In short, keeping the body healthy and clean, inside and out, helps prepare it to do the work of the spirit.

> *As we have seen, the expression of the spirit increases in proportion to the development of the body and mind in which it is encased. Therefore, yoga prescribes methods to train and develop the physical body and mind. The highly trained body must first of all be strong and healthy. The goal of all yoga teaching is how to concentrate the mind, how to discover its hidden facets, and how to awaken the inner spiritual faculties.*
>
> —THE COMPLETE ILLUSTRATED BOOK OF YOGA, SWAMI VISNU DEVANANDA

Traditionally, saucha includes such eyebrow-raising techniques as flossing one's nasal cavity with string, wherein a yogi guides the string up his nose and back down his throat, and irrigating the lower intestines in a manner similar to a colonic. The reality is that modern yogis have advanced levels of sanitation and self-care at their disposal whereas yogis living in India centuries ago were not so lucky. These practices originated as answers to a need for keeping the body clean and warding off possible disease. Some of their influences continue to thrive today, like the neti pot, for example, which many people swear by to alleviate nasal congestion. But there are other ways to apply the concept of saucha to our modern lives that have more profound effects on our health and happiness, ways of breathing a little easier that go beyond clear sinuses.

Eating clean is one of the simplest and best ways to keep your physical, mental, and emotional energy clear and balanced, as well as maintain a healthy body weight and prevent disease. Keep in mind that the foods we need most are marketed to us (and our children) least. Labels are purposefully misleading when it comes to ingredients. We all indulge on occasion—and a little indulgence can also be good for the soul—but when it comes to saucha's lesson of keeping the body clean inside and out, we must be mindful of the ways in which we nourish our body. Like a compass, saucha directs us back to feeling and thinking clean and clear when we veer off course. Ancient tradition didn't need to address diet. I believe modern yogis do because we have so many more options at our disposal. Let your diet be a daily ritual and celebration in balance. Have fun with your food; we're so blessed to have the options we do.

Other modern riffs on saucha might include little luxuries that help us clean up our proverbial act, feel fresh, and experience a spiffier outlook, such as a hot bath, pampering beauty treatment, or fabulous new haircut. This is the home of your spirit we're talking about! It's a privilege to treat it well.

Now that we've touched upon the home of our spirits, let's consider our actual homes, too. The Chinese tradition of feng shui harmonizes energy through how our environments are arranged, from which direction your bed faces, to keeping your desk uncluttered, to tying a pink ribbon around the doorknob to invite in new love (it can't hurt, right?). It's not yoga, but this other area of Eastern philosophy can have a profound effect on your personal space and energy. In *The Happiness Project*, author Gretchen Rubin chronicles a yearlong experiment of "trying to sing in the morning, clean [her] closets, fight right, read Aristotle, and generally have more fun," and discovers that a clean house is so important to happiness that it's the first chapter of her book. "Outer order contributes to inner calm," she writes. Which leads me to some of the easiest and most instantly gratifying yoga practices you can try anytime you're feeling weighed down, lethargic, or, well, quite frankly, like a mess:

- Declutter an area of your home that holds stale energy (think: junk drawer, mail pile, or closet). Attack it with spiritual ferocity, and then notice how liberating it feels to reclaim that energy and space in your life. After a major life transition, which included ending a long-term relationship and moving apartments, one lingering, miscellaneous box from my past remained in my new home. I didn't know what to do with it or wasn't ready to sift through the spooky relics and stray memories it might contain. When I finally did, it was miraculous. It was just one small box in one small city apartment, but once it was gone, I felt like I'd moved into the Four Seasons. It was *that* good. I felt spacious, free, and unfettered.

- Clean out the fridge and kitchen cabinets. If you don't want to eat it, it shouldn't be in your cupboards. Restock with whole foods, mostly vegetables in a vibrant array of colors.
- Splurge on your sanity by paying a little extra to detail your car, hire a nutritionist, or have your home professionally cleaned. Notice how this extra care and peace of mind affects the other areas of your life.

Once you master cleaning up your act, dressing the part of the lead role in your life, and creating conditions of outer order to inspire inner peace, it's time to step up your saucha game—to junky thoughts in your head and old cobweb aches in your heart. You can kick them to the curb, too. Picture bundling up grudges and leaving them for removal. Unclutter your heart: banish something heavy and unforgiven that's been collecting dust. Not because it's necessarily deserved, but because it's better for YOU. You're headed toward enlightenment—which means you need to pack light.

··

DO YOUR OM THING: BE IMPECCABLE

··

- What is one unhealthy diet or exercise habit I can clean up?
- What is one area of clutter I can clear out in my home?
- One junky thought pattern (known as a samskara) that I will throw out and replace with self-love. Examples: I'm not good enough, thin enough, rich, or smart enough, to name just a few.

··

Santosha: Contentment

I'm not sure who said, "Happiness is an inside job," but it's a great thing to remember as a yogi. *Santosha*, which means *contentment*, is the second attitude toward the self. *The Darshana Upanishad*, an ancient text with the purpose of uplifting the spirit (just think: Upanishads starts with "up"), also touches upon santosha, describing it as "delight in whatever fate may bring." Meanwhile, *The Mahabharata*, another sacred Hindu text dating between the *Upanishads* and the *Sutras*, calls contentment "indeed the highest heaven." No matter what the definition, the timeless message is clear: happiness is a skill and practice. Again, that's why yoga sees it as one of its self-restraints or forms of discipline. Happier people do not have easier lives, with less hard work, grief, divorce, or financial strain than the rest of us. They're simply more grateful for what they have and choose to be conscious of their contentment more often.

Modern yogis view yoga as a process of self-improvement. We do yoga so that we can get better at it. Gain greater flexibility. Become a kinder or more patient person. Excel at sports. Look better naked. The list goes on. In all the years I've practiced and taught yoga, I have never heard someone walk into a class and pronounce, "I'm here because I'm totally content with my life, body, and world view. There's nothing I seek to change or improve. I just want to learn how to do yoga, for fun." *Never.*

It's not that seeking self-improvement is bad. It's fantastic. The trick is to remember to enjoy the process. If we continually seek betterment, without a genuine appreciation for the present and "whatever fate may bring," we run the risk of missing the entire essence of yoga and, quite frankly, life. There is no fancy pose, enlightened style of yoga, venerable guru, or brilliant book that can manufacture or deliver your happiness. It comes from within you, and finding it is a different process for everyone.

When I demonstrate challenging yoga poses for my students, I often joke that no matter how impressive, graceful, or fun a yoga pose looks, it cannot change the quality of their lives in any major way. Performing a headstand won't save someone from getting a parking ticket, losing a job, or getting dumped. Meanwhile, the learning process, attention level, and attitude of the pose can have a positive compounding effect on the rest of our lives. Whenever you catch yourself hungry for the look and flash of an elaborate posture, remember your higher mission. Ask yourself if you're enjoying the process, not just flinging yourself toward an idealized destination.

When we forget that happiness is an inside job and look for validation externally—the house, car, or outfit—we will always end up disappointed. The house will never be big enough, car new enough, outfit in season enough. We'll lose the bigger picture of the process and fixate on the small stuff. Selfish stuff. Ego stuff. Want to know the shortest, most direct route out of ego? The opposite of the obnoxious voice in your head that says: *what about me?* It's santosha. It's gratitude. It's the skill of taking yourself out of the tailspin of scarcity and reconnecting to contentment. Because as soon as you put yourself in a state of gratitude (for anything, however small) you can no longer operate from ego. The two are polar opposites. The practice of santosha removes us from the rat race and rests us in a gentle hammock of gratitude for a little while. *Ahhhh.* Doesn't that feel better?

DO YOUR OM THING: NOTICE CONTENTMENT

- Keep a gratitude journal in which you write one to three things each day for which you are grateful. They can be incredibly small and ordinary: a warm house, someone who held the door, an email that made you LOL. Review the list before bed. Notice how this makes you feel.
- Think of someone in your life who seems to be deeply content. What do you think they might do to achieve that contentment?
- To unhook from a feeling of discontentment or ego, a funk or feeling of scarcity, Judith Lasater, cofounder of *Yoga Journal* and author of *Living Your Yoga*, recommends using the mantra: *how should it be?* Notice how your response to this question is an expectation. Not reality. If we are discontented with reality every time it does not go as planned, we lose the skill and gift of santosha.

Tapas: Discipline

Tapas, not to be confused with small tasting dishes in Spanish cuisine, are forms of heat or discipline used to control the body in the manner of an ascetic yogi. Ascetics are people who endure extreme measures of self-discipline by renouncing worldly urges such as delicious food, sex, outer beauty, and material wealth in the name of spiritual enlightenment. Often known as monks or nuns, they can be found in many faiths, including Christianity, Buddhism, Jainism, and Hinduism (in which case they are known as *sadhus*).

Ascetic yogis are identifiable in ancient art and contemporary photographs by their exceedingly frail frames, uncut hair or dreadlocks, and lack of clothing. If you hear of yogis sleeping on a bed of nails or walking over hot coals, we're talking about these guys. I still can't shake the memory of learning about ascetics in one of my favorite college courses, Sacred Arts of India, which surveyed yoga, art, and dance. My professor, Dr. Miranda Shaw, treated us to a slide show featuring yogis ascending to new levels of enlightenment through starvation, painting their naked bodies with cremation ashes, and hanging heavy rocks from their penises. Yes, you read that right. My male classmates howled. I averted my eyes, imagining a pain I'm not equipped to imagine. I was alarmed by how vastly different this image of yoga was in comparison to the gentle yoga I'd done with the senior citizens on Cape Cod or the serious Ashtanga classes I attended on Saturday mornings in a church basement off-campus. One could hardly help but think: *that is not yoga. That's insanity.*

Today our rituals are very different, but modern yogis still pursue an understanding of suffering and self-discipline. Part of our attraction to the most popular forms of yoga today—which are often physically vigorous and sometimes practiced in a sweltering hot room—is that they offer us a physical and mental challenge, a vehicle for self-mastery. They're hard, and, in bearing the difficulty, our bodies and minds become stronger. We steel our focus. I love this aspect of yoga and all forms of sports and fitness, for that matter.

When you're attempting a challenging pose that requires all of your faculties to be awake, nimble, and engaged in the moment, there's no time to indulge in illusion or distraction. For me, running offers a similar single-minded focus. We may not be treading hot coals like the sadhus, but we feel fire in our legs or lungs. We don't paint our bodies with ashes, but certain high-tech apparel makes us feel more impervious to the elements. A rock climber coats his hands in chalk. A ballerina tapes her feet. A swimmer shimmies into the latest, tightest speed suit before competition, a process that can take up to fifteen minutes and require the help of several teammates. Surfers don wetsuits like buoyant body armor for protection against the ocean's wrath. It's as though we're ritually covering ourselves in something for protection, whether physical or psychological. Then, we burn nervous energy, purge stress, and stoke the fire of our own endorphins through sheer physical effort. This is a healthy outlet. We're lucky for the proliferation of so many vigorous yoga styles over the years, stemming originally from Ashtanga. However, any well-meaning yogi or athlete can go too far, forgetting that we need to work in, as well as work out.

Furthermore, yoga teachings are careful to distinguish between using a level of effort, heat, or tapas to purify the body and senses and practicing asceticism to the point of ostentation or a "desire to win honor or fame." In other words, yoga's challenges are not for the purpose of showboating, and its mantra should never be "no pain, no gain." We encourage the quelling and control of desires and dis-traction but not making spectacles of self-deprivation. In today's terms, you might recognize this behavior among yogis who feel the need to advertise their too-frequent and emphatic juice cleanses or boast about how many yoga classes they take a week. It happens all the time. We start with a healthy habit, like drinking delicious, fresh juice, and take it to extremes. We've all done something like this at some point, but like the yoga path as a whole, we need to evolve to a new stage.

Sometimes, life requires an attitude of tapas: a fiery resolve, pointed strength, or sacrifice for a higher good. It's the part of us that needs to forgo short-term comfort for long-term growth and gain. It requires walking toward the burning coals rather than away. Ask an addict what withdrawal is like during the first days of detox, and the response probably sounds akin to sleeping on a bed of nails. Someone with low self-esteem or an eating disorder feels naked and exposed even when fully clothed. A modern yogi suffering from de-pression doubtless feels the heaviness of a boulder on his heart at all times. We all bear burdens, and we must summon the bravery and inner fire to face them instead of hide from them. We sometimes fall prey to mindless habits or self-destructive behaviors. We lose our way. We get lazy. We give up. Tapas lights the torch to guide us toward healing and home. Its purpose is never to destroy or deplete but to rebuild and reignite.

....

DO YOUR OM THING: LIGHT A FIRE

....

- In which areas of my life do I need more discipline?
- In which areas of my life am I making a show of my sacrifices or self-discipline?
- What is my bed of nails, heavy boulder, or hot coals? What step will I take to overcome this situation? Who can help me?

....

Svadhyaya: Self-Study

The ancient Greek poet Pindar once said, "Learn what you are, and be such," which eloquently characterizes svadhyaya, the yoga practice of self-study. According to tradition, two key ways to practice svadhyaya include reading books and reciting mantras. Again, we're reminded that unrolling a yoga mat isn't the only way to do yoga. It's one option, but there are many others. Reading this book might be your yoga for today.

For years, people have somewhat bashfully confessed that even though they don't really like yoga or practice it regularly, they enjoy reading my blog because it makes them feel "like a better person." "It balances the TMZ," a reader once told me. I love this honesty and don't think there's anything to be bashful about. Yoga, in any form, brings greater self-awareness, which makes the journey itself an accomplishment, whether we find ourselves on an inspiring blog, in the pages of a book, or on a yoga mat.

A mantra is a sacred sound, word, or phrase traditionally used to anchor the mind in meditation. You may be doing a riff on mantra meditation (known as *japa*) without even realizing it. *Om* is the most popular mantra used in yoga circles, and it has many interpretations. Most simply, it is intended to represent oneness, the sound of the whole universe, and interconnectedness of all things. It's the Divine vibration, the sound between sounds, the pulse of life itself. Mantras can be said aloud, repeated silently to oneself (as in meditation), sung in devotion (this is the practice of Bhakti yoga or Kirtan), or visualized in written form. I write them on my bathroom mirror in dry erase marker sometimes. My boyfriend really gets a kick out of this.

Beyond meditation, mantras are also very easy to incorporate into daily life, and you may find that once you start using them, the mind naturally gravitates toward the calming repetition of a favorite mantra when it needs a productive point of focus. They can soothe or energize our bodies in times of physical challenge; center our attention instead of letting it race in directions of anxiety; and connect our souls to the rest of humanity, God, or a higher power. The words of a mantra are less significant than the vibration they create—or the way they make us feel—when we chant them. It's the same reason we can love a song without knowing its lyrics or even understanding its language of origin.

A 2005 study involving veterans suffering from post-traumatic stress disorder found that their symptom severity, psychological distress, depression, quality of life, and spiritual well-being all improved significantly through the use of mantras. Athletes, too, often use key words to alleviate performance anxiety. In a February 2010 article called "Mind Games," world-class distance runner Kara Goucher told *Runner's World* magazine that she chooses a new mantra while training for each race. Words like "confidence" and "fighter" helped her maintain focus in grueling races at the 10,000-meter and marathon distances. Kara's coach and sports psychologist at the time were privy to her mantra choices. At key points in her races, her coach would yell her chosen word and watch it trigger a tangible result. She would bear down, find a new reserve of strength, and execute race strategy. The mantra helped transport Kara into "the zone," a coveted state during which an athlete's mind becomes clear, focused, and fully absorbed in the present moment. Yogis know this state as meditation.

DO YOUR OM THING: STUDY YOURSELF

- See the list of favorite mantras on pages 166–169. Choose one to integrate into your week. Use it to anchor your attention in meditation or yoga practice, repeat it while walking to work or folding laundry, or write it on a mirror in your home in dry erase marker.
- Think of a book that has inspired you or helped you discover an important truth about who you are. What was it? What did you learn?
- Ask yourself: What has yoga taught me about myself?

Ishvara Pranidhana: Surrender to God

For some yogis, the physical and spiritual elements of yoga coexist easily. But modern yoga often sacrifices some of its most important spiritual elements in order to make it palatable to newcomers. Examples of subdued spirituality include classes, teachers, and studios that omit references to God, imagery associated with the Hindu deities, or even chants of *om*. In fact, it's possible to practice yoga regularly for years, perhaps at a gym or with a teacher who prefers classes to be "No Om Zones" (a term coined by fitness-oriented teacher Kimberly Fowler), and never understand the spiritual foundations and practice of yoga. These environments are good for beginners who might feel uneasy about yoga's roots and meaning, but, like any path of learning or self-improvement, we eventually want to expand our awareness and level of understanding. We progress. People tend to sense yoga's spiritual element anyway because what they feel in class often transcends the purely physical. An essential element to acknowledging, exploring, or honoring the spiritual component of yoga and ourselves is called ishvara pranidhana (often translated to mean surrender to God). It doesn't mean we have all the answers. On the contrary, it means we surrender, with love, to the fact that we do not (cannot) have all the answers. Something greater is at work, and we can trust it.

In Chapters 9 and 10 we will address themes of spirituality and religion in greater detail, but to clear up any confusion in the meantime, the gist of the spirituality debate in modern yoga is this: yoga is a spiritual practice. It's not a religion. When the final niyama, ishvara pranidhana, asks us to surrender to God, it's not choosy about who or what God is. It reminds us that a higher power exists, and yoga can unite us with that higher power; however, your higher power can just as easily be a bearded man or a part-elephant diety, or the transcendent feeling of watching a sunset or holding a newborn.

Yoga is unconcerned with limiting, describing, or identifying God, and for our purposes as modern yogis, God (also known as the Divine, the Universe, Spirit, Universal Love, or Universal Soul, to name only a few terms) is any life-affirming force in which we have faith. Yoga asks us to have faith in God without requiring a specific image of it. Atheists, too, should not feel excluded by conversations about faith relative to yoga. A belief in the goodness of humanity and one's highest Self are also life-affirming forces cultivated by the practice. If the word or concept of God doesn't work for you, that's absolutely OK.

Through yoga, both on and off a mat, the yogi fortifies her spirit, one that is infinitely connected to the spirits of everyone and everything else. My friend and author Dave Romanelli has a wonderful mantra that he claims would make all of our lives easier if we could follow it: *Trust Your Journey.* I believe he's right. These three words are a beautiful, nondenominational, interspiritual example of the faith and surrender captured in ishvara pranidhana.

Trust. Your. Journey.

....

DO YOUR OM THING: HAVE FAITH

....

- Do I have a higher power, and what does it mean to me?
- When do I feel most connected to my spirit or best Self?
- Fill in the blank: if I had total trust in my journey, I would

  _____.

....

Limb 3: Asana | Practice

If yoga were the winter Olympics, asana would be figure skating. Summer Olympics? Swimming. If yoga were rock bands, asana is the Beatles. The Bard of literature. Monet to impressionism. Baryshnikov to ballet. It's the front row at fashion week and the recent discovery of the Higgs boson to physics. Asana is the headliner. It's what we know best, see most, and love the world over. It's the darling of the spotlight, where photographers train their camera lenses, and to the average observer, it encompasses yoga.

Except that it doesn't, which you've figured out by now. The postures are vitally important because they make us feel more vital and ready to do the larger work of the mind and spirit that yoga also encompasses. Or, as David Swenson, one of the country's foremost teachers of Ashtanga yoga, once said, "The paradox of yoga is that we use the body to figure out that we're not the body."

Asanas are mentioned infrequently in the *Yoga Sutras* and other ancient texts credited with formalizing yoga's framework and tradition, and their origins are debatable. This is largely due to the fact that yoga was an oral tradition for most of its history. Today, we know that some of the poses we do are very old (think: Lotus or Dancer's Pose). Ancient artifacts carved in stone of these postures exist and can therefore be carbon-dated with accuracy. Some are very new (think: anything called Flip Dog, Wild Thing, Rock Star, and the like). It's possible those are all the same pose. It depends on who you ask.

What we can all agree on is that the asanas give us something to practice. The word translates to mean *seat*, though today we use it interchangeably with *pose* or *posture*. Their realm is finite. Their instructions are clear. They teach us focus, perseverance, and patience. They yield flexibility, strength, and balance. "Practice and all is coming," Pattabhi Jois would famously say.

Entire books have been written on asana alignment alone, and many of them are masterfully done. I don't think I need to add anything to that genre, but a snapshot of my essentials includes the following advice:

- *Build a steady foundation.* Whatever is touching the ground (i.e., your hands or feet) should be steady and strong but not stressed or white-knuckling. Certainly there should never be pain. This is more common in kneeling postures or headstands, for example. The bottom line being that if the foundation is shaky or strained so is the rest of the pose. The structure is bound to crumble or give you a crick in the neck (possibly worse). It's also a wonderful lesson about our foundations as a whole. The footing on which we begin ripples through whatever we build—elegant yoga poses, trusting relationships, Jenga towers, you name it.
- *Stack your joints.* When in doubt about what goes where, think of stacking your joints. Just as the structure of a house is built from a sound framework, each stud meticulously placed, so are your bones and joints when you build asanas.

There are exceptions on occasion, but most often, think of stacking your joints in straight, level, long lines, knees over ankles and shoulders over wrists, for example. Strive for neutral and symmetrical alignment. In his book *Journey into Power* the great yoga teacher Baron Baptiste, for whom I worked directly for several years, explains, "You'll know when you've achieved neutral alignment in a pose when suddenly it ceases to be a struggle. You fall into a perfect relationship with gravity and you feel a sense of strength, stability, and overall balance."

- *Use your bandhas.* Some styles of yoga prioritize bandhas more than others. In general, the more vigorous the practice, the more important bandhas are. The term means lock, referring to an engagement of the pelvic floor (mula bandha, like a Kegel exercise); lower abdomen (uddiyana bandha, as if sucking in your belly to zip up a pair of skinny jeans); or throat (jalandhara bandha, as if lightly holding an orange between your chin and chest). Used alone or in concert with one another, the bandhas energize our bodies, improve posture, focus attention, aid balance, and even protect from injury. Uddiyana bandha is also the quickest weight-loss secret in the world. You want to lose a quick five pounds in a matter of seconds? Suck in your gut and stand up straight!
- *Invoke drishti.* Where the eyes go, the mind goes. Some styles of yoga give specific instructions for where one should gaze in a yoga pose (e.g., fingertips, belly button, tip of the nose). But anyone can relate to channeling energy through a focused gaze. This lesson, too, has a beautiful application to how we experience all of life. In short, what you look for, you will find.
- *Prioritize the spine.* Growing up on Cape Cod, a few of my childhood friends had fathers who were sea captains. We

called them "Captain" at home, and they shipped out for months at a time. As you can imagine, one did not goof off in those houses. Hell, no. There's a saying often found on ships or depicted quaintly on signs in beach houses, which goes like this: "If the captain ain't happy . . . ain't nobody happy." The same goes for the spine. Think of it as the captain of your asana's ship. Make sure it is as long and supple as possible, even when folding forward or bending back. Never place pressure on the cervical spine (neck) in particular. If you've slept awkwardly, and your neck feels funny, bypass poses that place any weight on your head, neck, and shoulders. (Poses to avoid include Shoulderstand, Headstand, and Rabbit, to list a few.) Remember, do not eff around at the Captain's house.

- *Focus on attitude over appearance.* The fanciful poses are fun. I love them, and you will see some of my favorites in the coming pages. In the beginning, they're the dangling carrot that keeps yogis going. And they teach useful lessons of tapas and persistence. However, we must be careful not to overprioritize outward appearances. This distinction is important for both our emotional health and physical safety. The "yoga" is not in the appearance of the asana but its intention and attitude. We use the body to see that we are not the body. We are developing the skill of being present with the moment, no matter what it entails. What would it say about us if we only wanted to be present for ourselves when doing something fanciful? *I only want to be with you when you look impressive.* That sounds like a death knell for any healthy relationship—with the self or anyone else.

- *Leave enough gas in the tank to get home safely.* It's no secret that yoga has gotten more strenuous in recent years. It's frequently melded with other forms of fitness, making it more desirable to a broader audience, especially one with limited

time and resources, needing a good physical workout and
anything else—meditative effects or spiritual enlightenment, to name two—is gravy. I tend to teach challenging
and athletically inspired classes, which encourage students
to explore and exceed their perceived limitations. Yet, the
mindfulness we hope to create in our asanas needs to extend until the posture is complete. Meaning: how we exit
the pose is *part* of it. We shouldn't hold something until
we're suffering to maintain it safely, and then collapse in a
heap on the floor. Not only is that potentially unsafe for the
body, there isn't much mindfulness in a heap on the floor.

There are no photos in the *Sutras* and no traces of alignment
points like those above, but what Patanjali does say about the practice of asana is rich.

Sthira sukham asanam.

Which translates to mean, "The pose shall be *sthira* [steady or
strong] and *sukka* [light or sweet]." In this simple thread we find the
essence of what we still aim to practice in every pose today. In a word:
balance. If we do this well, we exert the strength of muscles and the
force of our will but yield with lightness and allow room for sweetness. The fact remains that a yoga pose cannot change one's life in
any great way. It is the synergy of the whole practice and our attitudes
that change everything. So, the aim is to cultivate attitude over appearance. We do yoga poses for the life preparedness and presence
they build, how they make our bodies vital and minds sharp. Asanas
remind us that we get good at whatever we choose to practice. Yoga
asks us to choose our practices carefully, in our poses on the mat and
in our lives off of them. Luckily, the strength, courage, and power we
find in the former can follow us into the latter.

....

DO YOUR OM THING: PRACTICE

....

- Where is my strength?
- Where is my sweetness?
- How am I like my yoga practice on the mat?
- How am I not?

....

Limb 4: Pranayama | Life Force

The greatest miracle is that you are alive.
And one breath can show you that.
—THICH NHAT HANH

Most yogis immediately recognize *prana* as the way their yoga teacher refers to breathing in class; however, beyond the mechanics of inhaling and exhaling, expanding our lungs and contracting them, prana suggests something bigger and more powerful. "In sacred scriptures of Hinduism, for example, prana almost invariably signifies the universal life force, which is a vibrant psychophysical energy similar to the pneuma of ancient Greeks," wrote the late yoga scholar Georg Feuerstein. Likewise, this "life force," as it is commonly referred to, could be viewed as the same energy referred to in Chinese medicine and acupuncture as *chi*. The point is that there are many words to express this one unifying concept, much like the many names people have for God, a fitting parallel since the etymology of the word *inspire* includes the literal meaning *to fill with breath or spirit*. Traditionally, yogis believed prana to be the most important of the limbs, having the power to directly transport someone to enlightenment (*samadhi*). If reaching enlightenment via the breath

sounds far-fetched, know this much is certain for us all: breath is
the most important thing in our lives. It is our life. If something has
breath, it's alive. Life begins with our first inhale. Learning breath
control shifts our life force, alters our energy, and it's the most portable yoga and meditation tool available to us.

Think of it this way: you cannot take a breath in the past nor can you
take a breath in the future. Therefore, when you focus on a single ex-
change of inhaling and exhaling, you connect to the most important
moment in your life, the one that is happening right now. The present
moment. We have no influence over any other moment. Those behind
us are memories. Those before us are guesses. Learn to focus on your
breath, and you develop the power to simplify your life in a given moment and choose your conscious place in it.

Breathing purposefully helps to slow down our minds, calm the
nervous system, reduce stress, improve circulation, and give organs
a rest, among a host of other positive effects. "Yoga Breathing, Meditation, and Longevity," a 2009 study by R.P. Brown and P.L. Gerbag,
found that yogic breathing increases our resilience to stress and re-
duces anxiety, depression, and post-traumatic stress disorder. So,
breathwork not only improves bodily health, it also makes the mind
a more hospitable place to live. (The most consistent and inescapable
environment in which any one of us lives is our own head—talk about
valuable real estate!)

As a teacher, I often encourage students who feel particularly
overwhelmed or stressed on a given day to focus solely on their
breath: breathe deeply, and recite this mantra silently to yourself as
you do: I breathe in . . . I breathe out. Doing so trains the mind to
relax and return to the present moment. Like playing a musical scale
or balancing in Utthita Hasta Padagustasana, the more you do it, the
more skilled you become. You *can* simplify your life in a given moment. What's required is intention and practice. If lifting weights
makes your muscles stronger, think of breathwork and meditation as
workouts to strengthen your mind. So much of modern life compels

us to multitask and move faster. Yoga's power is in doing the opposite. The irony, of course, is that when you improve your ability to focus on one thing at a time, you increase your productivity for all things. Your efficiency, problem-solving capacity, and creativity are heightened manifold. Do less, and you become more. More inspired. More focused. More filled and fueled with prana.

In the pages that follow, I've detailed four essential *pranayama* exercises along with their energetic effects. I've arranged them from simplest and most portable (you can practice them on the subway or at your desk) to the most elaborate and even delightfully kooky, best saved for the privacy of your own home. Use them as needed, in combination with asana practice, or on their own.

Sama Vritti

(EQUAL BREATHING): *To calm and soothe.*

How to do it: *Sama* translates to "same," so the idea is to evenly match the length of your inhale to that of your exhale. For beginners, a three or four count is a good place to start. From there, you can work toward a five or six, then a seven or eight. If you're Michael Phelps, you can do several minutes. (Kidding.)

Ujjayi

(VICTORIOUS BREATHING): *To invigorate and focus.*

How to do it: Yogis of the Ashtanga, Power, and Vinyasa varieties have their Darth Vader breathing skills down pat. It's a thoracic breath (meaning it happens predominantly in the lungs, as opposed to the belly), which helps to energize the body during vigorous yoga practices. The belly lock (uddiyana bandha) is maintained while you breathe in and out through your nose, as you lightly contract the base of your throat. The result is that you will sound a little like Darth Vader or the waves at the beach. The translation of *ujjayi* is "to be victorious," which speaks to its strong, bold nature. I also love the image of it being a victory simply to take a moment and breathe this way.

Nadi Shodhana

(ALTERNATE NOSTRIL BREATHING): *To balance and create clarity.*

How to do it: Take a deep breath in through your nose and let it out easily through your mouth. Then, use your thumb to block your right nostril. Inhale slowly through the left nostril only and exhale slowly through the same side. Next, block the left nostril with your ring or pinky finger. Inhale and exhale through the right. Repeat for several rounds. Throughout the day, we rarely breathe evenly through our two nostrils. We always favor one. This style of breathing rebalances our breath and the two sides of our brain. Its effect is immediate and incredibly grounding. I even have the sense that I can see more clearly after I practice *nadi shodhana*, as if my eyes have been aerated along with my sinuses. (Note: you may want to blow your nose before practicing this technique.)

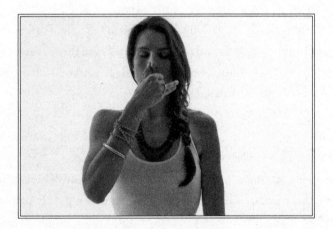

Breath of Joy

To energize and uplift.

How to do it: Get ready to let loose and feel as though you've had a shot of spiritual espresso! Breath of Joy is comprised of a three-part inhale through the nose and forceful exhale through the mouth.

Along with the three-part inhale, your arms will gesture like those of the conductor of an orchestra.

First inhale: lift your two arms together to the level of your navel.

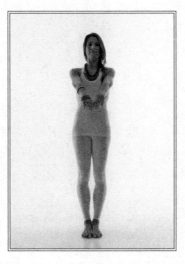

Second inhale: open arms to the level of your shoulders.

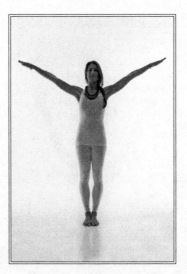

Third inhale: lift two arms together overhead.

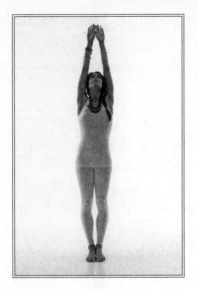

Now comes the fun part: like a downhill skier leaving the gate, throw your arms behind you as you squat down and breathe out your mouth, sticking out your tongue. (Repeat three to four times.)

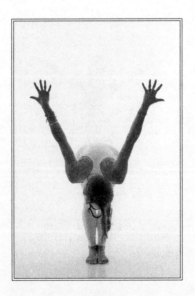

DO YOUR OM THING: TEND YOUR LIFE FORCE

- Choose one pranayama above and practice it. Are there times when doing this breathing exercise would help you more than your current stress response?
- Choose a small task you do regularly, such as answering the phone, turning the key in the lock, or flipping on the television. For one full week, take one long, slow, conscious breath before performing this activity. Notice how small increments of focus and breath can change your day.
- Spend time each day, on your mat or off, breathing as if it was the most important thing in your life. Because, actually, it is. Anything you hope to do or become begins with the fact that you are alive. You are breathing.

Limb 5: Pratyhara | Withdrawal of the Senses

On my thirtieth birthday, I disappeared. I wasn't trying to hide from the new decade that awaited me. On the contrary, I was excited about it. I'd heard good things, mostly from my mom, who raves about her thirties like they were a collection of charming islands in the Mediterranean she once visited. *I loooooved my thirties*, she reminisces. I probably would have gone to an island if time and budget were not constraints, so I went to a yoga and meditation center in the Berkshires instead, to see Deepak Chopra; some of his advice during this experience I mentioned earlier in the book.

I knew I needed a different type of birthday celebration that year—one that was quiet and reflective. I had been going nonstop for months (possibly years, maybe three decades . . . something many of you may relate to?), and my inner life needed time to catch up. So I escaped to a solitary meditation retreat in the mountains. Not completely solitary, of course. I was surrounded by hippie types and people who may or may not have changed their names more than once over the years to sound more Indian, exotic, or fully manifested, then changed them back again. I overheard a conversation in the café, where yogis have the option to indulge in coffee, sugar, or Wi-Fi not found elsewhere on the premises, between two people inquiring about a mutual friend, each updating the other on the latest name change to which they were privy. *But, what was it before that? And before that?*

When I began teaching yoga, I remembered feeling like a disappointment for having a last name so clearly ethnic but originating nowhere near Southeast Asia. By thirty, the tide had turned in my mind, and I was glad I kept my name, sparing family members and the post office the confusion. Retreat goers did yoga, danced, drummed, or chanted. Many wore clogs (myself included). I meditated, did yoga, ate vegetarian meals, put away my cell phone, and went to bed early. Privately, I craved sugar.

In the preceding year: I started my blog, often toiling on my laptop till the wee hours of the morning figuring out what I wanted to say and what on earth a widget was, and I ran my first marathon, regularly rising just a few hours later to train in frigid Boston temperatures at sunrise, before arriving to work long hours as a marketing executive at a magazine in the midst of a recession. I volunteered for favorite nonprofits. I was in a relationship, and we'd moved in together. I was busy. Life was full. I was mostly happy but privately seeking solace. Who was I if I stopped moving so fast? What was the essence of that "I" without all the ego trappings of work and striving? Who did I truly want to *be* in this new decade of my life?

The impetus for fleeing to the hippie hills on my birthday and running a marathon was the same: I needed to be alone. I craved quiet. I savored the simplicity of monklike regimentation: one foot in front of the other for miles upon miles while running, a curfew for lights-out, and silent breakfasts at the retreat center. Without realizing it, I was giving my yoga practice—no, my life—what it needed most: *pratyhara*, the withdrawal of our five senses.

During marathon training, I learned to enjoy running without music for hours at a time. When my running partner and I ran together each Saturday, we bopped along for miles of meaningful or mundane conversation or trotted close with scarcely a word. Cara was also on the cusp of thirty, getting married, and relocating to New York City all in one fell swoop. We had plenty to think and talk about, but sometimes, we preferred listening to our footsteps, turning them over like our thoughts, and listening inward.

Withdrawing our senses away from noise and stimulation and retreating inward has always been a key part of yoga practice, but it's even more crucial for modern yogis, who are subjected to exponentially more stimulus and lightning-speed connectivity at all times. Just as our ability to ramp up with adrenaline in times of danger (the fight-or-flight response) is an innate, biological gift, so is the need to let this surge of hormones subside. Because we're constantly living in an amped-up state of stress—even if it's the good, exciting kind, like marathons, big jobs, or growing families we're grateful to have—we *need* to unplug. Our minds resist, but our bodies desperately need the down time (our minds do, too, despite their protestations). When they don't get it, they start to rebel with a host of physical and emotional issues—the types of issues that land us in yoga classes to begin with and possibly the doctor's office down the road. It's estimated that 80 percent of all doctors' visits are stress related. Meanwhile, yoga and meditation practices, including pratyhara, turn off that agitating, mental fight-flight stress response.

Most of our energy is lost through our five senses, especially sight, each day. We spend our days looking, listening, smelling, feeling, and tasting things in the external world. These experiences can be inspiring, symphonic, scrumptious, soothing, and exotic—or graphic, cacophonic, disgusting, painful, and putrid. Each of our senses adds a layer of richness and depth to our lives. Yet, without care and cleansing, the combined onslaught can overwhelm and deplete us. Think about what the grating sound of a fire alarm or construction site is like all day or the feeling of staring at a computer until your eyes go blurry. The yogi learns to regularly retreat inward, to reset and reenergize.

Pratyhara is one of the most overlooked of the limbs—the one aspiring teachers miss on quizzes in teacher-training courses (if their teacher-training courses cover it to begin with)—yet its significance is more important for the modern yogi than any other yogi in history. Our senses, today, are assaulted at a much higher rate and volume than ever before, largely because of the Internet age. The smartphone age. The social media age. The age of on-demand and Netflix and exponentially more images per minute in the TV shows we watch, beginning as children. The more edits an editor makes, the longer the TV show might hold our rapidly decreasing attention spans. This is the age of potential, wondrous, technological distractions, if we desire, at all times. It's a fun time to be alive with endless options for how we allot our attention and communicate with one another, but it's also downright exhausting if we don't stop and turn our focus inward to recharge. Most of us are vigilant about recharging our cell phones and laptops each night. We know they have limited battery life. We are not so different. Turn off your sensory life on occasion. Plug in to your inner life. Both will be richer and more powerful for this practice.

Here are some easy examples for practicing modern-day pratyhara:

- Shut your eyes for a brief period of time during the day (i.e., not just while sleeping) and turn your gaze (drishti) inward, toward your heart or the inside of your brow (third eye). Ask yourself: who or what is doing the looking? This shift in perspective draws you inward, rather than only looking and focusing outward. The journey of the yogi is to go inward and know that deepest, stillest part of ourselves.

· Turn off all electronic devices for a period of the day, such as one hour before bedtime each night. Better yet, let your devices recharge in another room while you rest more soundly in bed—without the threat of buzzing or beeping and no chance of that little LED screen lighting up and disturbing your peacefully darkened boudoir. Artificial light at night interferes with our body's ability to produce melatonin, the hormone that controls the quality of our sleep. Suppression of melatonin has been linked not only to increased levels of sleep deprivation from which Americans now suffer but even more serious consequences such as increased risk of cancer, diabetes, obesity, and heart disease.

· If you always practice yoga with music playing or in a studio with mirrors, choose a quiet class without mirrors for a change. Fully focus your attention on your mat and yourself, without the distraction of outside stimuli. The true purpose of yoga is to quiet the mind, which should not be confused with the entertainment aspect yoga has taken on in recent years. Music is a "nice to have." It should never be a "have to have."

· Eat simply by choosing all-natural, whole foods and skipping sugar, caffeine, and strong spices for a while. This mild cleanse gives taste buds a rest. Soon, fruit tastes sweeter and you'll crave less sugar. Food will become a sensory experience again. Eating should be enlivening and joyful.

· Take a personal vow of silence for a half or full day. Communicate your intention to friends, family, and business associates (a weekend day is best for those who work Monday through Friday). Spend the time mostly in solitude, using as few words as possible. If you have a boisterous household, an occasional silent morning or silent breakfast is a nice way for the family to wake up mindfully and observe quiet together.

- Enjoy a walk or run in nature sans music or cell phone.
- Use an aromatherapy eye pillow during Savasana or other restorative yoga poses to draw your drishti (gaze) inward, rest your eyes, and soothe your olfactory nerve.
- Turn off the TV. A little is fun and relaxing. Too much saps our creativity; erodes relationships, which thrive on personal connection; deprives our minds of meaningful down time; and leads to more hours of inactivity each week. And there's no delicate way to say this: more couch time leads to more cushioning where you don't want it.

I turned thirty at the yoga and meditation center and met Deepak Chopra (who signed my tattered, dog-eared, underlined copy of *Seven Spiritual Laws of Success* and encouraged me to keep writing). After curbing my sweet tooth for a few days, getting some sleep, and getting off the computer, I packed up my car and headed down the winding and wooded roads toward the Mass Turnpike. I felt quiet, clear, and content. The leaves on the trees seemed to vibrate with new energy, their chlorophyll-hued edges crisply outlined by blue sky. *Had my eyesight improved from all the meditating?*

I stopped at a convenience store just before the highway and stood dumbstruck by all the colorfully wrapped, indulgent ways I could treat my taste buds after days of squeaky-clean eating. I opted to abstain. My brain felt too clear, my energy too steady, my body too light and open. I settled on water and almonds. When I got back into the car, I noticed an unfamiliar hush. I'd forgotten to turn on any music. Reaching for my iPod, I contemplated what I wanted to hear. Something upbeat? Rap? Electronic dance music? Stevie Nicks? I couldn't decide. I chose silence. I drove for a while basking in my preserved senses. My nerves weren't frayed. My eyes weren't tired. My ears were open. The multitasking death wish was gone. Eventually, I rolled down the window, turned on some music, and sang along—the sound of my happy, loud, off-key voice audible only to myself.

DO YOUR OM THING: TURN INWARD

- Which of my senses do I overstimulate?
- Power down all electronic devices. *Go ahead, you can do it.* And do not, under any circumstances, attend yoga class with your phone stationed beside your mat (unless you are awaiting a call from someone incarcerated, gravely ill, or you are a surgeon who needs to talk an intern through performing heart surgery while trapped in an elevator shaft).
- Create an Out of Office email message to increase productivity while working on projects that require unbroken concentration or to increase relaxation while on vacation. The manuscript for this book became its own yoga, and in order to finish, I knew I needed to stop spending energy in so many disparate directions. This was my solution. (If I owe you an email, I swear it's coming.)
- Download a productivity app, which can disable certain functions on your computer (such surfing the Internet, email, or social media sites) so that you can work without interruption.

Limb 6: Dharana | Concentration

For him who has no concentration, there is no tranquility.
—BHAGAVAD GITA

Think about the last time you were lost. Not emotionally, but geo-graphically. Maybe you were driving or walking in a foreign city or another part of your town, attempting to read a street sign, looking for the number of a building, or searching for a house. You needed to focus, so you turned down the music, got off the phone, and squinted your eyes a little to sharpen your sight. You honed your attention to-ward one, crucial task: becoming un-lost. This is dharana, or culti-vating the skill of concentration.

Concentration is the precursor to meditation, which means that if you have trouble meditating, you can start with concentration. In concentration, we focus on one object or task. In meditation, we be-come one with the object or task. It absorbs us. Instead of an experi-ence of *I am looking at that*, we feel: *I am that*. The Sanskrit translation for this phenomenon is *tat tvam asi*, which basically means that your deepest self, in its purest, primordial state, is the essence of every-thing else. I am the ocean. I am the air. I am the sun's warmth, the earth's solidity, the same as that bird, perched and watchful.

Before ascending to new levels of consciousness—or daily productivity—we must first learn to concentrate. A trained and fo-cused mind is the most potent force in the world; therefore, dharana maximizes, balances, and restores mental energy. Through the de-velopment of one-pointed focus, the mind becomes disciplined to take in less extraneous information and align with the most essential information in a given moment. There's less clamor and more clarity.

You may recognize that there is an element of pratyhara needed to successfully practice dharana. We need to tune out certain sensory distractions in order to concentrate. This skill aids us in balancing on one foot on the yoga mat, sinking a putt on the golf course, finishing a work project under a tight deadline, or looking intently into the eyes of a loved one who needs our undivided attention. In a culture hell-bent on giving everyone or convincing everyone that they have an attention disorder, dharana is a remedy. (This is not to say that pharmaceutical remedies are bad, only that they are often overprescribed and abused.)

Strong concentration has physical implications as well, including the capacity to perform tasks requiring enhanced agility, endurance, speed, or precision. Asana, athletics, dance, and other forms of movement are key examples. One instance in which dharana came to my rescue occurred in the early days of training for my first marathon. Overjoyed by the news that I had officially decided to run, my speed-demon friend, Jennelle, suggested we should spend some quality time together while she was visiting Boston over the holidays. I would have been cool with a cup of tea or a bite to eat, but Jennelle insisted on running nine miles in the freezing cold, up Heartbreak Hill (the most-punishing section of the Boston Marathon course, which is actually comprised of four hills in succession).

The roads were slick with ice, and passengers in oncoming traffic peered out frosty car windows to gawk at us, a gaggle of women dressed like Alaskan fishermen with all our layers of clothing, barely any skin exposed, barreling downhill (*finally*) toward Boston. Temperatures dipped below zero that night, and public-service announcements warned people to stay indoors. Our sweat froze into icicles in our hair beneath our winter hats. The cold air seared our lungs. Windy tears stung my eyes. And that wasn't the worst part.

The worst part was that I couldn't keep up. (Does anything sting more than the ego perceiving imminent failure?) The group bounced ahead, while I plodded behind—slow, freezing, and scared.

The gap between us widened, with Jennelle hanging back as much as she could. I winced with guilt: running slower meant more time in the cold for her. I cursed myself for not thinking to bring emergency money for a cab. I started to panic. If I couldn't hack the last nine miles of the course, I certainly wouldn't be able to run the entire 26.2.

Thank god, dharana kicked in to save me. I started watching Jennelle. Really watching her and nothing else. I fixed my eyes on her back—my strong, unstoppable friend—and willed myself to keep her within eyesight and footfall. She'd run at least one marathon per year for the past seven years, raising tens of thousands of dollars for cancer research. She knew these streets. She'd weathered this cold. She could pull me, I thought. I visualized a rope between us, as one towing a distressed vessel ashore. As long as she charged forward, I could follow, I told myself. I stopped worrying about the pace, temperature, icy roads, looky-loos in cars, or the class of photography students in Kenmore Square now snapping photos to capture the coldest night of the year. I have no idea if they got a shot of us running by with less than a half mile to go, but for me, the snapshot in my mind remains. Even with its reputation for breaking hearts, Heartbreak Hill did not get the best of me that night. I made it home, not by the strength of my legs so much as the strength of my concentration. Because what is life and the experiences we craft within it other than a result of where we focus our attention?

Cultivate your powers of concentration with the following real-life practices:

- Spend five to ten minutes contemplating a single image, such as a candle, favorite piece of art, photograph, holy card or statue, mountain, or flower. (If you struggle with meditation, this is an excellent first step.)
- Schedule an hour of reading and allow your attention to be fully absorbed in a book.

- Make a point to look at everyone with whom you speak, with the same attention you give a close friend.
- Enjoy your favorite music, TV show, website, crafting project, or whatever else you relish on its own, rather than diluting your attention across more than one of these pursuits simultaneously.
- In yoga class, fix your gaze on a single point in every pose. As a yoga teacher of mine once said: *You shouldn't notice what the person next to you is wearing. Unless your long-lost brother or sister walks into class, you do not look up.*
- In standing balances, remind yourself that the point of the asana is not balancing on one leg, it's focusing the mind on one task at a time. Try a new, more challenging standing balance for one month.
- Isaac Newton famously wrote, "If I have seen further, it is by standing upon the shoulders of giants." To this end, don't be afraid to let others help you see beyond your own abilities. Teachers, coaches, parents, siblings, partners, and friends are perfect people from whom you can borrow focus and vision to elevate yourself to new heights.

....

DO YOUR OM THING: IMPROVE CONCENTRATION

....

- Think of a time when you experienced unbroken, laserlike concentration. How did it feel physically, mentally, and emotionally? What were you doing? How can you do more of it every day?
- When are you best able to concentrate? Think about the time of day and surroundings and whether you're in solitude or with others. How can you best take advantage of these times?

- What mental images help focus your mind and energize your body, such as a special spot in nature, "spirit animal," or personal hero?

....

Limb 7: Dhyana | Meditation

What I have to say about meditation boils down to this: it never hurts. It always helps. It costs nothing, and it improves everything. There are so few things on earth of which this can be said. Not prescription drugs (side effects). Not therapy (costly). Not red wine and chocolate (temporarily improves outlook, nay waistlines and inhibitions). Yet, many modern yogis are still intimidated by sitting still and focusing on the moment. Not because they don't want to, but because they are convinced they're *bad* at it.

We lament that we'd *like* to meditate. We know the benefits—from reducing stress, to improved immunity, to changing the body's chemistry from the inside out beginning with the brain—but we're not capable of the fundamental skill required for meditation, which is the ability to *stop thinking*. We've tried. We sit cross-legged. We close our eyes. We breathe deeply. We anticipate peace, clarity, and enlightenment, and, instead, we get: *I'm hungry. What time it is? My nose itches*. We write mental grocery lists and to-do lists. We daydream about the person we want to date or marry or the ex we wish would rue the day he or she left us. We wonder about the weather forecast. We visualize a chic outfit from a wardrobe we don't actually own and then feel dejected that we don't own this outfit. We hate our job. And our boss. No, not our boss. She is nice. We want pizza for dinner. Sound familiar?

The problem is that this logic is flawed. The purpose of meditation is not to stop thinking. That's impossible. The purpose of meditation is to observe our thoughts and develop the strength to unhook from them, to see them for what they are: passing and impermanent. The mind's natural tendency is toward movement and fluctuation, recreating moments in the past and racing toward speculations about the future. It's not wrong, bad, or a sign of meditating ineptitude. It's simply the way the mind works and a gentle reminder of how infrequently we are fully present in our daily lives. Herein lies yoga's biggest gift: the ability to reconnect and wake up to who we truly are. I'll give you a hint: we are not our outfit for tomorrow or desire for pizza tonight. The thinking mind won't stop altogether, but we can find space between our thoughts, and in this space, we find our deepest selves.

It will always be tempting to fidget, flee, or Facebook update instead of inhabiting the present moment, which can be challenging and uncomfortable, even tragic and terrifying, at times, but it's this lack of consciousness that leaves us feeling like we need yoga in the first place. The feeling of missing our own lives, as they are happening. For the modern yogi, the mat is the place where he/she goes to address feelings of disconnection: from the self, our health, what we feel, who we are, and who we want to be. If life feels busy, complicated, crowded, or lonely, a yoga mat offers the opposite. Yet, the asana practice addresses who we are from the outside in, and unless we can get to the root of what distracts or distresses us and let those distractions go, things will not change much. Meditation is so central to the practice of yoga and feeling whole that four of the eight limbs relate to it in some way.

Meditation is the natural, graceful state of being yourself and knowing who that is. When we are fully absorbed in the present moment, paying attention *on purpose* and *without judgment*, we are meditating. This is the definition offered by one of my favorite meditation teachers, Jon Kabat-Zinn. So, set aside all previous failures and frustrations. Disregard the belief that you're too busy or anxious. Stop waiting for a guru. Allow yourself the freedom to *be*, without judgment. Watch your thoughts, feelings, and sensations without reactivity. Befriend your Self. Rest assured that you already know how to meditate. You just need to begin. And remember, the only way that you can be bad at meditation is by not doing it.

....

DO YOUR OM THING: MEDITATE

....

- Turn to Chapter 8 to learn more about different kinds of meditation. Choose one style and practice it for ten to fifteen minutes a day for one week. What do you experience?
- Remember, if meditation is too difficult, you can always scale back to concentration (dharana). You can focus on a mantra. You can focus on your breath (pranayama). You have so many tools already!

....

Limb 8: Samadhi | Enlightenment

Let me be clear: I am not an enlightened being. Not a guru. Not even that good at Scrabble. I study yoga, as I have for many years, and I've been teaching what I know since before I was legally old enough to order a glass of wine. My students from that time forward have achieved all kinds of personal and professional fulfillment with yoga as a cornerstone. But none of this means that I can unlock the secrets of the universe for you, let alone myself. And even if I proclaimed to be an enlightened guru, I couldn't tell you whom to marry, whether you should get an MBA, attend culinary school or sign up for yoga teacher training, or who will win the next Superbowl. That's not enlightenment. That's fortune-telling, which is entertaining in movies but not very reliable in real life. True enlightenment, on the other hand, is real.

Yoga teaches the most important kind of reliability one can find: the kind you have on yourself. Like Dorothy in *The Wizard of Oz*, who had the ability to return home to Kansas whenever she wanted, yogis have enlightenment (sometimes called superconsciousness) within them all along. The beginners, unwittingly wearing socks to their first class; the sophomores who revel in each increasingly intricate posture; and the veterans, compounding yoga's positive effects over time, feeling inspiration wax and wane but still staying the course: enlightenment exists within each of them already. This deep and meaningful connection to Self or the Divine—since we're all glints of the same spark—culminates in a state of supreme bliss and higher consciousness. It is the ultimate goal of yoga and final limb: samadhi, which literally means, "to stand inside of," as in you, standing within your Self, in full possession of its truth and brilliance. Yoga does not manufacture or create it. It only reveals a light that's been there all along.

Look, there it is. There you are.

Our instinct is to think of enlightenment as counter to or elevated from ordinary life, but the opposite is true. Heck, my Yogi brand tea bag once told me "When you know that all is light, you are enlightened." Not bad, little tea bag. Not bad at all.

In his book *After the Ecstasy, the Laundry*, author Jack Kornfield talks about the profound experience of elevated consciousness for several modern yogis; once they became enlightened, they still had to address the mundane realities of daily life, or as Kornfield wrote: "Although the experience is special, it does not happen to a special person. It happens to any of us when the conditions of letting go and opening the heart are present, when we can sense the world in a radically new way." The words of Mahatma Gandhi, invoking the source of enlightenment in each of us (referred to as God or Spirit for some), remind us, "If you do not find God in the next person you meet, it is a waste of time looking for him further." Characteristic of her beautiful book *The Art of Doing Nothing*, Veronique Vienne explains, "You are not a perfect being, but your mind is clear. The charade is over. The painful existential headache is gone. At long last, the unexceptional seems extraordinary enough." In other words, you and your daily life have the power and conditions needed for enlightenment, and yoga offers the tools for this realization. I may be enlightened after all, but so are you. Various styles, teachers, and techniques provide access and inspiration, but they are not the source of samadhi. The source is in you. Getting there is your om thing.

His Holiness the fourteenth Dalai Lama is not a yogi in our contemporary use of the word (you won't catch him in Crow Pose, and he absolutely does not wear stretchy pants). But he is certainly a teacher and example of many of the yoga principles and practices discussed so far, including samadhi. Twice I've spent time in his presence, which profoundly influenced my understanding of what enlightenment is, what it looks like, and how anyone might get there.

For "His Holiness," for short, or "HH the DL" for shorter, enlightenment was determined for him at the age of three by a spiritual search committee. After several auspicious signs and a series of tests, the committee decided he was the reincarnation of the thirteenth dalai lama. For the rest of us, the process is very different. We're not charged with being the spiritual or political leader of a country as toddlers. We try to live fully into our own being, the best way we know how. Enlightenment is not about learning airs or affects, becoming a monk or perfect yogi, it's about regaling your life with realness and compassion.

It's about embracing your karmic role in the world, however you see it. The Dalai Lama is a holy person, the most visible Buddhist in the world, spiritual leader of Tibet, former head of state of Tibet, a monk, scholar, winner of the Nobel Peace Prize, and, to some, a reincarnated saint (the bodhisattva of compassion, Avalokiteshvara—thirteen dalai lamas ago). As a result of the Chinese occupation of Tibet in 1959, His Holiness has lived in exile in neighboring India, spreading his message and light around the world, becoming a kind of spiritual rock star. As I've mentioned earlier, the studies of yoga and Buddhism are not the same, but they are complementary philosophies in many ways, arising in nearby geographic locations several thousands of years ago. Today, they continue to influence each other.

"It was like the man carrying the lamp left the room," John F. Kennedy Jr. once said of the moments after His Holiness departed following one of their encounters. This reaching across cultures and faiths to affect people is the hallmark of this particular dalai lama.

Before, during, and after my experiences of seeing His Holiness in person, I've thought a lot about what it means to be our own incarnations of peace. I've contemplated enlightenment, as yogis see it, as Buddhists see it, as I see it. This is what I've learned:

- *If people are laughing, they're listening.* Of all the exceptional things one notices about His Holiness, his laugh is chief among them. It bellows. It's contagious. It makes people glow and giggle and forget, if only momentarily, that life is also filled with sad, serious things about which we cannot laugh. It would seem, then, that enlightenment carries an element of lightheartedness.
- *There are no throwaway moments.* I watched the Dalai Lama retrieve his glasses from a cloth satchel midway through a lecture on the Four Noble Truths, and it took a painfully long time. Elegantly long, really. I think he forgot we were there. All ten thousand of us. He wasn't fazed by people anxiously watching and waiting for his speech to continue, bothered by the minute task, flustered or bashful that he didn't locate them sooner, or in need of a handler to do it for him. Most of us would bumble apologetically, our cheeks flushing in front of all those watchful eyes. I'd likely give up and suffer without them. What I realized is that there wasn't anything more significant for him than getting his glasses in that moment. It was *that* clear. The

most important moment of your life is the one that's happening right now. That's an enlightened way to live.

- *Negativity is largely mental.* The Dalai Lama is adamant about this, and given his ebullient persona, you'd be hard pressed to doubt him. He says, "90 percent of all negativity is mental." Which isn't so groundbreaking, but we all need reminders. Change your thoughts; change your life.

- *We're all the same.* "Everyone has the desire to have a happy life," he told us. "We are the same: 100 percent. Same." Consider the magnitude of that statement for a moment. If we could all live by it, it would revolutionize and remedy so many issues of inequality and social injustice.

- *Compassion is essential to happiness.* This is the magic of seeing him in person. The compassion is palpable. No gesture tossed away. No laugh conjured for show. He does not seek to impress. He exudes peace and love but makes no demonstration of either. His language is direct. Like the rest of us, he's vulnerable to cold and wind, sun and heat. I perceived no filter between who he is and what he does. If he was cold, he paused to drape his robes more snugly around his body. If the sun glared in his eyes, he rifled through his few material possessions to find tinted eyeglasses. He's simple but never sanctimonious. He knows a lot but isn't all-knowing.

- *Tune inward.* When asked, "What's the one, single thing that we can all do to promote peace, His Holiness exclaimed, "I don't know! Things are too complex; there's no single thing." The crowd collectively laughed (again). It's pretty liberating to have a holy man tell you he doesn't have it all figured out, either. Enlightenment is not omniscience, he reminded us. There is no easy fix, no magic bullet, no elixir for the reality of the human condition and the state of our world, which is often riddled with hardship, violence, and injustice. We're all in this together, and everything we do affects everything else. When life is painful for one of us, the rest of us are God's grace. When asked how he might advise young people today, he advocated greater self-inquiry and reflection, instead of constantly distracting ourselves through sensory stimulators, such as TV, cell phones, music, and more. At this, he even pantomimed putting headphones into his ears. Tune inward, he was saying. In other words, practice pratyhara. Stop fleeing the moment and your Self in favor of quick comforts. Look inside. Pull up a chair in the quiet room of your own mind and learn to be comfortable there. Find happiness there. If you can't, you will not find it elsewhere.

Nothing the Dalai Lama says teaches samadhi as much as his way of being. No word, phrase, or speech can capture enlightenment. Instead, I saw it when he rose to leave. Better yet, I felt it because it silenced an entire stadium. I even caught the moment on video. It's unremarkable footage, but the remarkable reveals itself. An old man slowly gets up to exit. He bows to the thousands of people watching; he mindfully says farewell to the other monks on the stage, and he leaves. No one speaks. No one moves. A person coughs in my vicinity. Everyone is transfixed.

The word for enlightenment, *samadhi*, is the same for both yogis and Tibetan Buddhists. The Chinese call it *wu-wei*. The Japanese say *satori*. In Hebrew, it's *d'vekut*. We know it when we see it, yet it's hard to describe. It's the moment when the internal struggle stops, the battle with what is inevitable: what *is*. Being is enough. The mind is lucid, open, and alert. The world's problems haven't ended. We still have scars and wrinkles. We still get parking tickets on occasion, and they gall us (the key is, hopefully, not for long). We are ourselves, and this knowledge is, for a change, a source of ease.

....

DO YOUR OM THING: CONTEMPLATE

....

- Which moments each day are you throwing away? Remind yourself that they are real and significant. No matter how mundane, your journey, spirit, and best self are in those moments.
- Practice a form of yoga or mindfulness every day, whether it's a yoga class (*asana*), breathing exercise (*pranayama*), or a few moments spent in silence, prayer, or meditation (*dhyana*). Time with yourself, noticing the details of the experience of the moment, is the best way to feel awake and alive.
- Think of an enlightened being, someone you know personally or, perhaps, a historical figure about whom you've read: what aspect of this person inspires you? What about the nature of life do they illuminate for you?
- Imagine that you have experienced samadhi. What would this enlightened version of who you are tell the current you? Tell yourself this anyway.

Part Two

The Body

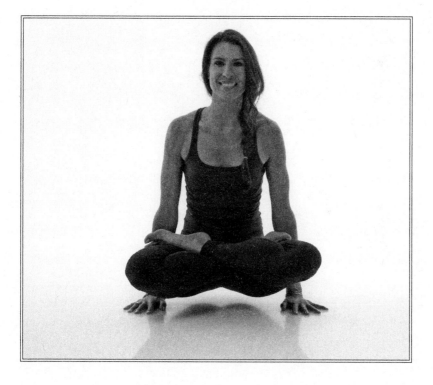

CHAPTER 3

What Do You Want to Embody?

I am often asked—by yoga students, readers of my blog, media types, even casual acquaintances at dinner parties—what the secret is to getting a *yoga body*. In fact, here is a brief list of some of the most commonly asked questions that I get about the yoga body. Scratch that—the most commonly asked questions I get. Period.

Will yoga help me lose weight?
Are you vegan?
Have you heard of this juice cleanse?
Are you gluten free?
Have you heard of that juice cleanse?
What do you do for cardio?
How often do you run?
Which yoga poses will strengthen my core?
And lift my butt?
Do you do Pilates?

What do you think of CrossFit?

Do you lift weights?

Do you wear a heart-rate monitor or wearable fitness tracker?

Should I do a juice cleanse?

I enjoy the fact that people trust me enough to ask me these questions, and I'm delighted to (forgive me) weigh in on their queries. Helping others to become more healthy and mindful is validation for me that I'm doing work I'm meant to do.

But my favorite piece of advice is the same for everyone, and it has nothing to do with explicitly choosing a type of yoga, fitness trend, diet, or cleanse. It's about choosing a mind-set or, possibly, a heart-set. Because the truth is that it's not about *what* you do, but rather, *why* you do it.

If yoga means to *yoke* or *join together*, what is it, exactly, that we're joining together? One simple answer is: the body, mind, and spirit.

The Subtle Body

If we didn't know better, it might be easy to assume that the practice of yoga is solely concerned with the physical body—specifically, how it looks and performs. But of course this isn't an accurate portrayal of the ancient mind/body practice, nor is it the most effective approach to personal wellness today. As you've gathered, our focus in this section of the book is on the yoga body—how we define it, care for it, and experience its whole potential and health through yoga, in our own way. But, by way of a spoiler alert . . . the physical and spiritual pursuits of yoga are inextricably linked. By definition, yoga is about their connection and synergy. And, the good news is that if you do yoga, you have a yoga body. Hooray for that!

The reason that talk of the yoga body gets muddled is because few people are actually referring to the body as it relates to the tradition and practice of yoga. Instead, the yoga body is defined by what we read in magazine interviews or how *some* bodies look in photos. We see a feature with Jennifer Aniston or Gwyneth Paltrow, lithe and limber, skin and hair glowing with some kind of ethereal beauty. *She does yoga. That's a yoga body*, we think. We want that. Who can blame us?

We temporarily forget that looking at an image could never be confused with what it feels like to be that person (no matter how lithe or beautiful), and a retouched body ideal reveals little of the power of yoga practice and how it can truly make someone glow from the inside out. Of course, vigorous asana practice will certainly help you attain some version of the coveted *yoga body*. It will make you strong and flexible, able to balance or possibly fly (à la arm balances), but making this our primary focus is a major buzz kill for the experience of yoga—and authentically being yourself. The benefits of yoga are not available to us when we look a certain way. They're available to us as we are, right here, right now. Yoga offers what you need to feel whole and, yes, beautiful, in a variety of ways, only some of which are physical.

So what I want to explore here is a more thoughtful and holistic perspective, as yoga tradition would have it—including an explanation of the subtle body with its seven *chakras* (energy centers) and five *koshas* (layers). Through this ancient method made modern, we'll create our own approach to looking *and* feeling our best. To begin, I'll share the best piece of yoga body advice I can offer to anyone who asks. It's not a pose or style of yoga, workout tip, or trend. It's more of a mind-set. Heart-set, actually, because the intention behind anything colors everything. Instead of focusing on how you look, identifying yourself by diet, or grasping for the latest trend, think about this one essential question:

What do you want to embody?

Seriously. Think about it. Because the answer will be telling, and the actions needed to achieve this state will become easier to identify. If you know how you want to feel, you'll make better choices about how to get there.

For instance, you don't want to embody artificial colors, flavors, or feelings. You don't want to embody scarcity and deprivation. If you want to embody strength or confidence, aligning yourself with yoga teachers, fitness regimens, or diets that promote diminishment or depletion won't get you to your goal. If you want to feel joyful and light, you can't choose workouts that are drudgery or engage in self-talk that is demoralizing. Sure you can lose weight on a certain diet, cleanse, or workout regime, but will you *feel* light? Will the weight loss last? Or, will it dissipate—like anyone's capacity to stay on a diet or regime forever? If you want to *embody yoga,* you must learn to pay attention to the gift of your life in a single moment—even if it's a difficult moment. Do this by listening to your life force, your breath. If you want to embody speed or endurance, your workouts must prioritize the same. If you want to feel energetic and endorphin-drunk, then you've got to get up and move like your life depends on it (because it does). If you want to embody beauty, you'll have to do things that genuinely make you feel beautiful. They are not usually available in stores. They frequently include smiling or laughing. Remember: mind-set. Heart-set.

The ways in which we choose to move our bodies and nourish ourselves are two of the greatest gifts we are given every day. The best wellness resource at your disposal is one you already have: your mind. Changing the body starts with changing the way you think. Begin with what you want to embody, and let that word, feeling, or mantra dictate the choices you make, on the mat and off.

Embody grace. Eat energy for breakfast. Run with heart-pumping, leg-burning, soul-exhilarating speed. Balance with confidence. Breathe with love. Put on your clothes with joy. Take them off with acceptance. Embody yourself fully. It's a beautiful thing.

What Is a Yoga Body?

When I began to write this book, I also started teaching Do Your Om Thing classes in Boston. They're not held at a yoga studio but, rather, at an adult education center, where the smell of culinary classes wafts in from a state-of-the-art kitchen down the hall and the sound of verbs being conjugated in French echoes nearby. Most participants in my DYOT class arrive directly from work at the end of a long day, wearing business casual attire as opposed to yoga pants. It's a welcome change for many, as we have the opportunity to close the gap between how yoga is done on a mat and how we practice it in our lives. After the course, my students leave knowing more about yoga philosophy and tradition from our hours of talking, reflecting, studying, and sharing than they might after years of *asana* practice. Most of all, they immediately possess new ways of practicing yoga in real life as opposed to merely on a mat.

Like this book, the course is separated into four sections relating to yoga philosophy and the yoga body, mind, and spirit. The first major shift for students relates to this conversation about how yoga views the physical body.

For fun, I pose the question: *What is a yoga body?* I write this question on a whiteboard and ask the group to call out whatever comes to mind first. *How would you define it? What does it look like? Who has one? What does a yoga body eat?* (The answer to this last question is unanimously kale, followed closely by quinoa.) The body brainstorm is a fun and eye-opening exercise. People immediately shout the obvious descriptors: *thin, bendy, sweaty! Little shorts! Shiva Rhea! YOU!* Nonphysical qualities are thrown in, too, such as calm and peaceful, but these are dwarfed by the abs and asses that students disproportionately see in the media and supermarket aisles.

Once we have a robust list, I ask another question: is it possible to meet the given criteria—to look like a prototypical yogi; be sweaty,

bendy, and thin; eat lots of kale; wear tiny shorts—and still be a raving lunatic?

Answer: yes. Absolutely.

Yoga studios are crawling with raving lunatics. We all know at least
a few. I'd venture to say we've been these raving lunatics at least once
(myself included). Outward appearance made not a bit of difference,
did it? If you want balance, if you want to feel a sense of peace in your
life, if you want to experience yoga and true connection to Self, you've
got to do more than wear teeny shorts and eat kale. It's time to walk
the walk, right off your mat and into your life—real life—not some
blissed-out yoga unicorn dream, not your life after teacher training, a fancy retreat, getting married, being promoted, or losing five
pounds. The gift of doing your om thing is that you do it right now.
Coincidentally, *now* is the very first word of the first yoga sutra, in
which Patanjali wrote, "Now, begins the yoga." All these centuries
later, we still begin with now.

After the initial brainstorm, the class explores the body according to yoga wisdom, including the chakras and koshas of the subtle
body. We reflect, meditate, chant, journal, and break out into smaller
groups and pairs for discussion. I try to keep it aboveboard, not too
hippy dippy, and most of all fun. Students use what they learn and
combine it with what they already know—a wealth of life experience
as busy people trying to find balance in a fast-moving world. Our
exploration starts where most yoga classes end, literally and figuratively.

CHAPTER 4

The Chakras:
Feeling Light from the Inside Out

The word *namaste* closes most Western yoga classes today. It means *the light within me bows to the light within you*, and yogis interpret this light in myriad ways. You can think of it as the inherent goodness within each person, a spark of the Divine or Universal Soul in each of us (known as *atman*), or a glow radiating from the "wheels of light" known as *chakras*, the seven energy points residing within your body along the spine. The challenge is to honor this sentiment in our lives without sounding too precious or ending up like Russell Brand's character in *Get Him to the Greek*. While hurling horrible insults at each other, his movie ex-wife, played by Rose Byrne, blithely trails an offensive remark with namaste, as if the latter were capable of inoculating the former. "You do not get to say namaste to me right now!" Brand's character rants. He has a point. Nice yoga words are hollow if our actions do not align with what we say. It's better to focus on inner intentions and how they emanate outward.

According to yogic literature, chakras (pronounced with a *ch*, as opposed to *shhh*) are wheels of light or bundles of energy housed within our bodies. Think of them as traffic roundabouts (to New Englanders: rotaries) for the energy in your body. At best, these confluences of energy—both in the body and on paths out of it—optimize efficiency. At worst, they create serious traffic jams. Traditional yoga wisdom sees traffic jams in the chakras as sources of illness and disease within the body. For instance, stuck energy in the heart chakra could present itself as blocked arteries, leading to heart disease. While modern science offers us a more detailed understanding of the body, this ancient system of thought still provides wisdom for modern yogis about how we can best care for our physical and psychological health.

The chakra system includes seven major points of energy (there are smaller ones, too) located along the spine, from your tailbone to the top of your head. If you're skeptical that there's a meaningful energy point on the top of your head, go to a swanky hair salon and get your scalp shampooed and massaged into a sudsy lather. When the stylist reaches the top of your head, pressing firmly, and all the tension in your entire overstimulated, jumbled brain ceases, there's a strong possibility you'll become a believer. For yogis, the crown is said to be the home of enlightenment or superconsciousness, which might explain why I swear I've heard angels sing when my head is in one of those salon sinks.

Each of these bundles of light and energy corresponds to aspects of your anatomy, psychology, spirituality, and more. They're not physical masses that would show up in an X-ray but intersections of energy through which we experience our bodies and the world around us. Tending to or ignoring these invisible parts of your body influences how you look, feel, age, and address illness or imbalance.

With that said, here's a brief explanation of each chakra, what it means, and the best ways to keep its energy bright and clear. Some of these strategies will be brand-new and some familiar. It's possible that you've gravitated toward certain chakra-balancing strategies on your own simply because they work, which is the only endorsement you need. If it works, if it makes you feel lighter, it's part of your thing!

The Subtle Body: Light and Layers

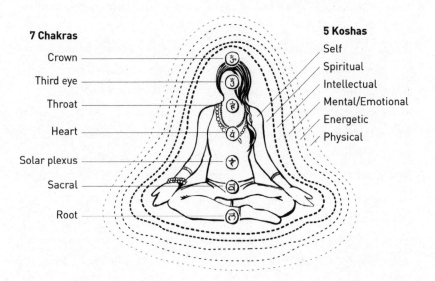

7 Chakras
Crown
Third eye
Throat
Heart
Solar plexus
Sacral
Root

5 Koshas
Self
Spiritual
Intellectual
Mental/Emotional
Energetic
Physical

Chakra 1 | Root (muladhara)

The root chakra is located at your tailbone, and its extensions include your legs and feet. Its purpose is to ground you. It's your base. It represents who you are and whom you trust. Its desire is survival and stability. It says *I belong here.*

When you sit on the floor in meditation or stand firmly planted in your feet and legs in Tadasana on a yoga mat or in your boss's office while asking for a raise, you are connecting to your root chakra. When you dash around frantically, attempting to do too many things, in too many different places, at the same time, you lose this connection. You're temporarily uprooted.

Imbalance in your root chakra manifests as the frenzied feeling that precedes leaving your keys in the doorknob overnight, putting your sunglasses in the refrigerator, or accidentally driving away with your wallet on the roof of the car. You don't know whether you're coming or going. You might feel unsafe or unsure about a major relationship or aspect of your life. The rent is due. The laundry pile climbs. The thought of dealing with that stack of mail, its utility bills, the expiring this or that, makes your skin hot and prickly. It's become hard to make plans because you don't know where you want to be today, let alone in two weeks, or two months.

When the region of the first chakra is out of whack, it can cause physical dysfunctions such as increased anxiety; poor sleep; pain in the feet, knees, legs, or buttocks; lower intestine issues (such as constipation); immune-related disorders; eating disorders; and more. Ultimately, you should see a doctor for medical issues, but this way of viewing the body can help to develop a more preemptive and holistic picture of your health so that you can be more proactive in managing it. Psychologically, a lack of stability and security from not knowing *where you stand*, as it were, are first-chakra issues and killjoys for intimate relationships. Without feeling grounded and safe in who we are and whom we trust, it's pretty hard to have close bonds, trusting relationships, intimacy, or a fulfilling sex life (which becomes even more pertinent to the second chakra, as we'll learn a little later). Alternatively, when you feel rooted in who you are, understand your basic needs and personal constitution, have people in your corner whom you trust, and have your house in order (figuratively or literally), then you experience innate pleasure, a greater ability to concentrate, and delight in the boundaries that make you feel safe and, ironically, free. You have roots, a base, a sense of home. Or shall we say hOOOMmme?

Paying rent, buying groceries, or raising children who go to bed on time and stay in their beds (as opposed to climbing into yours and depriving you of sleep) may not sound sexy, but creating boundaries and meeting our basic needs help create a sense of grounding and security in our lives. How divine a full night's sleep feels after it's gone missing for weeks, months, or years. From a grounded base, we're more open to life's natural joys, including but not limited to healthy expressions of sexuality and sensuality, which also originate in the lower region of our bodies. Meanwhile, ending a long-term relationship, getting a divorce, or being in debt, for example, can make us feel insecure, scared, or stuck. These negative feelings represent first-chakra issues, too.

Things we can do to balance our root chakra run the gamut from surefire tools for feeling more bold and badass (how you want to feel when you stand in your boss's office readying to ask for a raise) to subtler practices that have cumulative effects over time. All serve the purpose of shifting the energy at the base of our bodies. For example, wearing the color red—which is associated with this chakra— may boost our mood or raise our energetic frequencies. Perhaps you've heard that women wearing red can elevate a man's heart rate more than any other color or that red cars get pulled over more often. This color is powerful, so why not use it to your advantage? Color therapy isn't necessarily yoga, but it can unequivocally influence the energy of your body. Think about your favorite colors: which ones do you typically wear? Which ones do you use to decorate your home? Consider how people express unity by wearing school colors, team colors, or colors associated with political or social causes. Using color to express emotion or signify connection are things we do naturally. Partly because we crave connection; it is human nature and the nature of yoga. Wear red and connect to your powerful root chakra.

After the Boston Marathon bombings and harrowing week that followed, culminating in a citywide lockdown during which we were told not to open our doors for anyone other than uniformed police officers, people in Boston felt unhinged to say the least. I don't mean to retell a news story you already know. What I want to tell you about is what happened as the news trucks departed.

We went outside. We savored normalcy. We grocery shopped and walked our dogs. We took kids to the playground and said thank you to police officers in the streets. Still shaken and stunned, we were trying to sink our roots back into the earth.

I visited a growing memorial at the finish line, blocks from my home, piled with flowers, notes, American flags, Tibetan prayer flags, candles, religious mementos, and lots of sneakers. I noticed how quiet it was and, among other details, what people were wearing. It was as if our mayor had sent a memo: *Wear blue or red for our country or beloved Red Sox* (who went on to improbably win the World Series a few months later, transforming from a last-place team into a first-place one). We also found a mantra to signal our unity and support for the victims: *Boston Strong*.

Another powerful practice that can immediately work within the present structure of all our lives—however busy—is the use of mantras, which I touched upon earlier and will revisit in greater detail when we talk more in depth about meditation. The mantra that supports the first chakra is *lam*, which you can chant like *om*. If Sanskrit isn't your thing, you can simply say the words *I am* to yourself. Let this be, perhaps, the one time and place in your day when you don't have to fill in the blank. Instead of: *I am a yogi. I am a parent. I am a teacher. I am a CEO.* You get to just *be* and feel connected to your innermost and infinite Self. Settle into that stability and trust in your own being. Here, *I am.* I belong.

In the book *Eastern Body, Western Mind*, which offers a more comprehensive interpretation of the subtle body, author Anodea Judith likens the chakra system to our own personal constitution, reflective of our basic rights. Associated with the first chakra is the right to be where we are and have what we need. Whenever you feel out of place, lost, marginalized, scared, or made to feel small: stand or sit up straight. Plant your feet. Take a deep breath. Tell yourself: I AM. Be grateful for all that you are, even if it means you don't have all the answers. Know that you belong—to a legacy of yogis, a family, a community, a city, most of all, to yourself. You don't need to change. You need to root and reconnect. The fact is nothing can uproot, unhinge, or oust you from your sense of self, unless you let it.

ROOT CHAKRA ESSENTIALS:

- Intention: I AM
- Mantra: Lam
- Color: Red
- Focus: Grounding, security, creating healthy boundaries. Basic needs such as food, shelter, and safety.
- Asanas: Standing poses (such as Warrior variations), standing balances, seated poses, and forward bends. Supta Baddha Konasana (Reclining Bound Angle Pose) is a relaxing option when life feels extra frantic (shown using props).

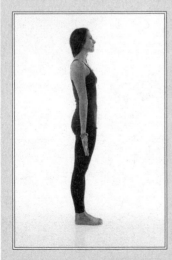

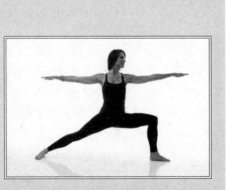

Tadasana
(Mountain Pose)

Virabhadrasana II
(Warrior II)

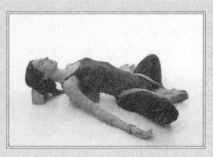

Supta Baddha Konasana
(Reclining Bound Angle Pose, variation with props)

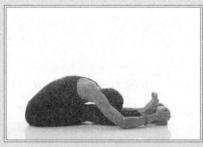

Paschimottarasana
(Seated Forward Bend)

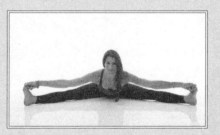

Upavistha Konasana
(Wide-Angle Seated Forward Bend)

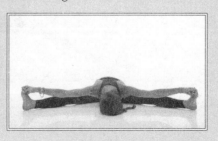

Chakra 2: Svadhisthana | Sacral

The second chakra is located in the lower back and abdomen. Think of this as the home of your creativity, whether you're creating art, building a business, or growing a baby in your womb. It's where you feel butterflies when you're excited or queasy when you're nervous. It's a fierce and intuitive energy hub in the body, and, today, greater scientific evidence suggests that the gut is so complex that it serves as a second brain.

Dr. James Greenblatt, a Boston-based psychiatrist who specializes in treating eating and mood disorders through integrative medicine explains, "There are more neurons in the GI tract than anywhere [in the body] except the brain." He keeps this discovery in mind when he treats patients, some of whom come to him as a last hope after seeing many other doctors and trying many medications. In the case of one young patient suffering from severe OCD and ADHD, Dr. Greenblatt homed in on imbalances that other doctors had missed—not in the patient's mind but her stomach. He added probiotics (beneficial bacteria for the gut, found in many cultured and fermented foods) to her treatment program, which also consisted of therapy and medication, resulting in an almost complete cessation of her symptoms within six months. After one year of the probiotic prescription, there was no sign of her ever being ill. So, it seems the ancient yogis were onto something. The region of the lower abdomen is incredibly powerful and intelligent. It can offer important cues for keeping the rest of our bodies balanced and healthy. To talk about "gut instincts" or having "a fire in one's belly" invokes—anecdotally and scientifically—the second chakra.

Our gut is also thought to be the home of our inner drive (hence terms like "gutsy" or "gutless"). I have a friend who perfectly articulated this aspect of the svadhisthana chakra without even realizing it. While also working full time as a marketing executive at *Runner's*

World magazine and raising two small children, she managed to qualify for the Olympic trials at the marathon distance. When we met, I marveled at her ability to balance working full time, raising a family, and running at the highest level of competition. I assumed she must have had a lot of practice over a lifetime of being an elite competitor, accustomed to juggling athletics, first with schoolwork, then career, relationships, family, and motherhood. Turns out, I was totally wrong.

"I didn't start running until I was twenty-seven," Kathleen told me. I figured she must have played a sport in college, maybe soccer. Running would have built upon the speed she already possessed. She shocked me when she said, "I was never a runner. I wasn't athletic. I didn't even like gym class."

Wait. What?

I was dumbstruck. It's one thing to pick up running at age twenty-seven, something to stay in shape, maybe do a 10K with friends. But to discover you've had a latent Olympic-caliber gift waiting to be unleashed your whole life? It must have been like opening your mouth to sing in the shower and realizing you sound like Beyoncé. (Never mind, that's a bad example. Everyone thinks they sound like Beyoncé in the shower.) You get the idea, though. One day, my friend Kathleen went out for a jog, and not so many days later, she was chasing down an Olympic dream.

"What was it like?" I asked.

"Like someone lit a fire inside me," she replied.

"Fire in the belly," she calls this kindled inspiration. She even has the Japanese character for the element of fire tattooed on the right side of her lower abdomen. It has nothing to do with chakras for her. She'd never done yoga before we met. But in the language of yoga, this inner fire is her svadhisthana chakra. Its color is orange, which is appropriate for the warmth and light our creative embers and instinctual gifts bring us. In an anatomical sense, your lower belly emanates a lot of heat. If your hands ever go numb from the cold, an outdoor leadership guide might tell you to take off your gloves, unzip your coat, and put your icy hands in contact with your belly. It isn't fun, but it works.

The second chakra's mantra is *vam*, or you can focus your attention on the words I FEEL, without being judgmental or ashamed of what shows up. Just say *I feel* and, then, listen for what comes next.

It sounds simple, but, for many of us, it takes years to realize that knowing how we feel is a prerequisite for creating the life we want. This realization stands in stark contrast to thinking you want a certain prescribed outcome for life—a job, marriage, or lifestyle you believe you *should* want—without honoring how it makes you *feel*. How many fewer midlife crises or divorces would there be if people truly listened to what was going on inside themselves before committing to careers that don't light them up or partners who don't make them feel anything but deeply loved and loving? Imbalances of the second chakra can include lower back pain, menstrual irregularities, digestive problems, hormonal issues, sexual dysfunction, and more. Ignoring, suppressing, or swallowing the emotions we feel is a sure way to stress or sicken this region of the body.

One day when Kathleen and I were having a technical conversation about proper running form, she told me, "You have to lead with your belly button, like something is pulling you from there." I smiled at the image in my mind of the second chakra pulling her forward.

SACRAL CHAKRA ESSENTIALS:

- Intention: I FEEL
- Mantra: Vam
- Color: Orange
- Focus: Creativity, pleasure, movement, gut instincts.
- Asanas: Hip openers, such as Half Pigeon or Frog Pose, lower abdominal strengtheners, and lower back stretchers.

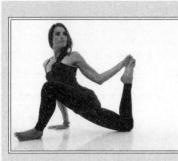

Utthan Pristhasana
(Lizard Lunge, variation)

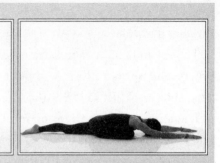

Eka Pada Rajakapotasana
(Half Pigeon)

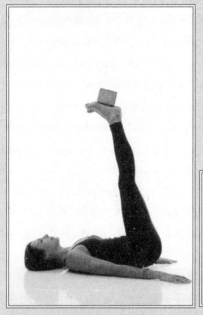

Lower Ab Isolation
(block optional)
Isolate your lower abdominals
by lifting and lowering your
tailbone off the floor, or
pretend to write your name
on the ceiling, using your
abs to steer your feet.

Reclining Half Pigeon

Chakra 3: Manipura | Solar Plexus

If you were to thrust out your solar plexus like a superhero, you'd access the location of your third chakra; it's the space above your navel and below your ribs, referred to as the solar plexus for the complex network of nerves radiating from this literal center of your body. Think of it as the home of your ambition and courage. I picture the Cowardly Lion finally full of gumption and standing proud. It's where you take a heaving deep breath before taking a plunge of any kind. It's standing in Warrior II Pose, squaring your ribs and shoulders directly over your hips, arms extended like wings, feeling open, capable, and strong. A spiritual six-pack, if you will.

The sound associated with this chakra is *ram*, which sounds a lot like Ra, the sun god of ancient Egyptian religion. It's interesting to notice cultural, linguistic, and symbolic similarities among ancient civilizations. The first yogis were part of one; the Egyptians were another. When their stories, sounds, or symbols overlap, many people believe it suggests a greater connection or universal truth in play across time, place, and culture.

The color of your third chakra is a bright, golden yellow. Here, you summon your power to act. You know who you are, thanks to your first chakra. You know what you feel because of listening to the gut feelings in your second. Now, you know what to do. You take action. Your mantra is I DO. When this chakra is balanced, you have steady metabolism, easy digestion, and willpower in spades. You can stick to a diet, stay off cigarettes, or kick a pesky Internet addiction. When it's off-kilter, it might manifest emotionally as a lack of self-esteem or excess of ego or physically in adrenal issues, intestinal problems, arthritis, diabetes, eating disorders, chronic fatigue, and more. The personal constitutional right of your manipura chakra is to be free.

One simple way to experience your third chakra and revive its power is to do a simple breathing exercise:

- *Place your hands on the bottom portion of your rib cage with your longest (middle) fingers touching at the tips.*
- *Take a giant breath and feel your fingertips pull apart as your lungs expand. Notice how empowering this feels.*
- *As you exhale, feel your ribs melt (tension, too). In Pilates, this action is known as* knitting *your ribs together. Your fingertips will touch once again.*
- *Repeat this pranayama, noticing the expansion and contraction of the area around your solar plexus chakra. Imagine its sunny, yellow color and the healthy furnace of your metabolism and digestion. Get reacquainted with your willpower, ambition, and courage.*

SOLAR PLEXUS CHAKRA ESSENTIALS:

- Intention: I DO
- Mantra: RAM
- Color: Golden yellow
- Focus: The power to act, individuality, and courage.
- Asanas: Sun Salutations, upper abdominal strengtheners, twists, and any poses that make you feel courageous and ready to conquer fear (arm balances, anyone?). Twists of all varieties, including seated, standing, reclining, and prone, are known to be detoxifying because they cleanse organs and increase circulation. They're also great for the spine.

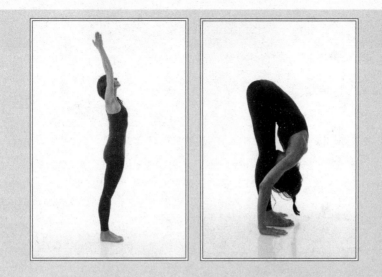

Urdhva Hastasana
(Mountain Pose
with Arms Overhead)

Uttanasana
(Standing Forward Bend)

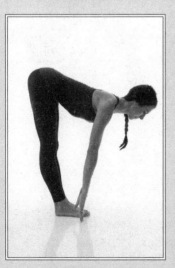

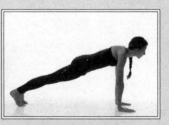

Ardha Uttanasana
(Standing Half
Forward Bend)

High Push-up
(also known as Plank)

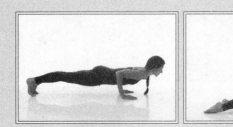

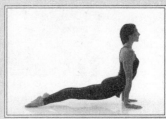

Chaturanga Dandasana
(Low Push-up)

Urdva Mukha Svanasana
(Upward Dog)

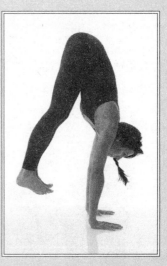

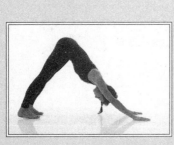

Adho Mukha Svanasana
(Downward Dog)
Walk or jump to the top of the mat and repeat
Standing Half Forward Bend, Forward Bend,
and Mountain Pose to close.

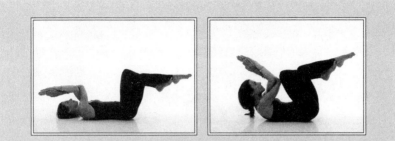

Eagle Sit-ups
Inhaling, reach your fingers and toes away from each
other. Exhaling, crunch your knees and elbows together.

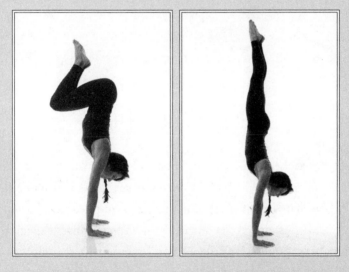

Hand Stand Tuck   Adho Mukha Vrksasana
                            (Hand Stand)

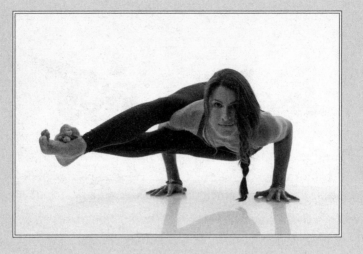

Astavakrasana
(Eight-Angle Pose)

Chakra 4: Anahata | Heart

For all the clichés you've heard about following your heart, there's only one thing you really need to know about yoga's verdict on them: they're true. The importance of listening to your heart isn't woo-woo nonsense. It's essential to your health and happiness, especially in relationships. Understanding and embracing this principle is also the difference between practicing yoga to cross an item off your to-do list and experiencing it in your life. I know because I've conducted extensive research on the subject. By which I mean I learned the hard way: by *not* following my heart.

We've all done it at some point, and the key is to learn from the lack of listening. Through yoga, life, and the yoga of life, I figured out what was blocking my heart. I'll save you the suspense: it was fear. Always is.

The heart chakra can experience balance or blockage, and we

certainly know that it can break. It can mend or stir with a word, song, or smile. It flutters at countless things. For some, it's Mozart. For others, it's Ryan Gosling. None of these experiences can be cajoled or manufactured. When Confucius implores, "Wherever you go, go with all your heart," or Shakespeare writes, "Go to your bosom. Knock there. Ask your heart what it doth know," this is what they're talking about. They may not have been yogis, but they understood the language of the heart. The heart speaks to us constantly, and it is our job to listen. The *Chandogya Upanishad*, a foundational yoga text dating back as far as 800 to 500 BCE, before the *Sutras*, tells us:

> *There is a spirit that is mind, life, light, truth, and vast spaces. It contains all actions and desires, all perfumes, and tastes. It enfolds the entire universe. This is the Spirit [Atman] that is in my heart, smaller than a grain of rice, or a grain of barley, or a kernel of a grain of canary-seed. This is the Spirit that is in my heart, greater than heaven itself, greater than all these worlds.*

Which seems to capture the same sentiment of Walt Whitman, when he famously wrote, "I contain multitudes" in his "Song of Myself." Each of us contains a heartfelt song or spark of the soul of the whole universe. We're filled with possibilities and passions known only to us, until we set them free in the world through our actions. Finding the heart's inspiration and authentic voice is what ancient yogis sought thousands of years ago and modern yogis seek now. It's the purpose of this book—to close the gap between what's happening on your mat and what's happening in your heart. "This is a subtle truth: whatever you love, you are," wrote Rumi. Therefore, you not only love yoga, you *are* it. In the same way that you don't find true love outside yourself; you connect with someone who ignites a part of you that's been there all along.

The anahata chakra is located in the middle of the chest, governing the respiratory, circulatory, lymphatic, and immune systems. Like all chakras, its light radiates forward *and* back—an important reminder for us to listen closely to our heart's deepest desires and humblest murmurings. Burying feelings in the back of your heart leads to imbalances, including but not limited to shortness of breath (e.g., panic attacks), upper back or shoulder tension, high blood pressure, or heart disease. The word *dis-ease* itself illustrates what the heart lacks: ease. When your heart feels broken, hopeless, or uneasy, it can be helpful to ask for *ease of heart* and set this as an intention for your meditations, yoga practices, or morning walks with the dog. This intention shifted things for me when my heart space started feeling like a run-down junkyard. I didn't have answers, but I knew I needed to find ease. We all need a little extra at some point, whether for getting out of bed in the morning, saying I love you, or sitting with ourselves and knowing deep in our hearts that we are enough.

Like all stages of yoga practice, the first step for transformation is awareness. I recommend this awareness-building meditation to do almost anywhere to improve your ability to listen, heal, and live from your heart.

- *Sit comfortably, and close your eyes.*
- *Feel your spine lengthen; imagining all your chakras in alignment, from your tailbone, connected to the floor (or a chair), to the top of your head, reaching to the sky.*
- *Place one hand in the middle of your chest and cover it with your other hand. Notice your heartbeat.*
- *Take a big breath in. Feel your heart rise into your hands, and, then, exhale all the breath out, every trace of it. Do this a few times.* Now, listen to your heart. *Especially at the base of the exhaled breath, before you inhale again. It's very quiet there. Just listen.*
- *You will be amazed by what you hear when you decide to connect.*

This skill is vitally important to your health and happiness. If you listen to your heart enough, it becomes harder and harder to act out of alignment with it. It becomes easier to find and create its highest good. It makes weighty decisions more nimble and heaviness in your chest lighter. In addition to the heart meditation, you may also try other fourth chakra–balancing techniques such as listening to or creating music. As a traditional yogi, this would include Bhakti or devotional chanting, to uplift the heart. As a modern yogi, it might include blaring and belting out your favorite power ballad.

The color associated with this chakra is a rich, vibrant green, like emeralds or parsley. As a holistic nutritionist and author of *UnDiet*, Meghan Telpner likes to say, "Eat color and wear color." Greens in particular are great for keeping your ticker healthy (and skin luminous). Go to a lush, natural landscape (the opposite of a run-down junkyard) and breathe its vibrant energy right into the middle of your chest. The mantra for your anahata chakra is *yam*, or you can repeat the words *I love*. Maybe your heart will fill in the blank, listing the people and life experiences you love. Or, you will only need the gentle reminder that you, the subject, enact the most powerful verb on the planet. *Whatever you love, you are.*

Most of all, balancing your heart chakra requires you to surround yourself with people you love, who make you feel whole and alive. Remember that *love feels loving*. Remove or limit exposure to those who make you feel small or toxic. Do the types of yoga and physical exercise that exhilarate you and make your heart pump. Practice backbends, the physical expression of being openhearted. Find a career that more often than not makes your heart sing, because it is your professional calling or gives you the stability and flexibility to put time and energy into your personal calling. Travel where whole hearts have gone or lived before you. Read poetry. Spend time with children, who have no trouble living from their hearts. Read some more poetry. Look at art. Laugh at comedians. Open your heart chakra to all of it.

HEART CHAKRA ESSENTIALS:

- Intention: I LOVE
- Mantra: Yam
- Color: Green
- Focus: Love, compassion, gratitude, forgiveness.
- Asanas: Chest openers and backbends. If love were a yoga pose, it would be a backbend, offering your heart to the world. Backbends can be energizing and exciting but also scary, like love itself! Here are three stages of backbends for anytime your heart needs a little lift (or a big one), along with poses to strengthen and support your chest, shoulders, and upper back.

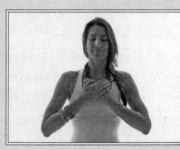

Heart Listening

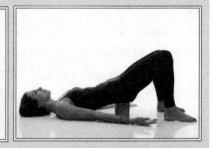

Setu Bandha Sarvangasana
(Bridge, supported
variation on a block)

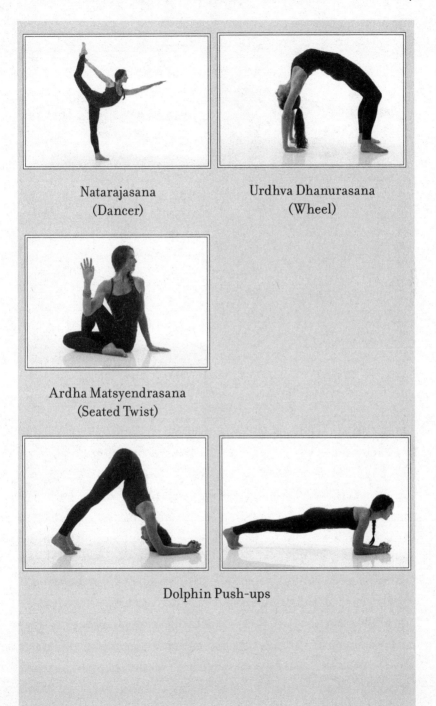

Natarajasana
(Dancer)

Urdhva Dhanurasana
(Wheel)

Ardha Matsyendrasana
(Seated Twist)

Dolphin Push-ups

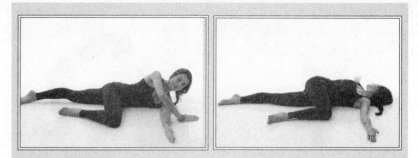

Prone Twist

- Pranayama: For the heart chakra, in particular, pranayama has a soothing effect, since it includes the respiratory system. Sama Vritti is a simple breathing exercise (see page 54) to do anytime.

Chakra 5: Vishuddha | Throat

Building upon the heart below it, the fifth chakra is also crucial to our happiness as yogis in the world and in relationship with others. This chakra is the home of our communication and self-expression. It's known as *vishuddha* and is comprised of the throat, neck, jaw muscles, and thyroid. Conditions such as laryngitis, chronic sore throats, teeth grinding, and neck tension originate in the throat chakra. Like the heart chakra below it, which loves music, the throat chakra also responds deeply to sound, specifically by creating it through speech, song, or mantra.

The idea that what we say is part of being a yogi sometimes escapes us. First, because making noise isn't customary in most yoga classes, save for a few *oms* to start and conclude a practice, perhaps an occasional sigh when something feels good, a guttural grunt when something is effortful, or the rare comment or question for the teacher or a fellow yogi nearby. Second, we're human. Once we're off our mats and in the world, we sometimes say things we don't mean. We let our emotions get the best of us. We judge others harshly. We're careless with the lasting impact our words can have, flippant with their gravity. We may even figure that as long as the person about whom we're speaking unkindly doesn't hear us, it doesn't count (i.e., gossip). The energetic system of the chakras and ancient wisdom of the subtle body don't buy this. If we say the words, we've created their energetic vibration in the world. Even if we're the only ones who hear the negativity, it has an effect. The language of our words, spoken and unspoken, profoundly affects who we are and how we feel, physically, mentally, and emotionally.

The field of body language research is a fascinating example of what happens when modern scientific discoveries support and validate ancient yoga principles. Positioning the body in postures of yoga or meditation has long been thought to impact the mind. Today, experts can measure changes in the brain after holding a certain body position for as little as two minutes. Social psychologist and Harvard Business School professor Amy Cuddy gives a powerful TED Talk on this topic. In her speech, "Your Body Language Shapes Who You Are," she outlines the practice and benefits of "power posing" or using the body to express desirable qualities, such as warmth, confidence, and competence—exactly how you'd like to feel before a job interview or while speaking in public, for example. Through what she calls a "free, no-tech life hack," Cuddy shares how to positively alter both the energy you exude to others and chemistry felt within your own body by increasing levels of testosterone, the hormone that emboldens us, and decreasing cortisol, the hormone that makes us feel stressed (among other negative effects).

The activity is simple but the results are profound. Power poses are defined as those that take up space, such as standing with both feet firmly planted on the floor, hands on hips, chest open, and the neck elongated and exposed. When we feel confident, we take up space. When we lack confidence, we cower, close off, hunch, and shrug. In fact, I've noticed that all the power poses have something in common: an open, unguarded chest and throat.

Not long after seeing Cuddy's TED Talk, which has garnered more than eighteen million views as I write this, I spoke at a wellness conference along with body language expert and author of *You Say More Than You Think* and *You Can't Lie to Me*, Janine Driver. Driver's area of expertise is in reading body language and training personnel in government agencies like the CIA and FBI to do the same while interrogating criminals. Again, a key piece of her advice homed in on the vicinity of the neck and throat. As an exercise, she had all the conference participants turn to one another and pay a compliment while protecting their necks in some way (stroking their throats, tugging at the collar of their shirts, or holding the side of their necks). "Do you believe each other?" she asked. The answer was a resounding "no."

Meanwhile, exposing the throat is a sign of confidence and trustworthiness. Driver even offered the tip of elevating the chin slightly by holding it in one hand—seen as a symbol of intelligence and power. "Chin to win," she called this gesture, while displaying photos of power players such as Oprah, Hillary Clinton, and Bono all striking this affable and assertive pose. No matter how you evaluate this theory, as a yogi or social scientist, via body language or yoga practice, the message is loud and clear: being conscious of how you express yourself, verbally and nonverbally, makes you more present and empowered.

The color associated with the vishuddha chakra is light blue or turquoise, a sky palette that inspires the airiness associated with speaking openly and freely. After all, vocal cords produce sound by conducting air. Before you give a speech, have an important conversation, or tell someone you love him or her for the first time, turn your attention to this chakra. Say the words *I speak* to yourself or chant the mantra *ham*. Both yoga and speech are forms of expression. Make them clear and true. Do Fish Pose, Shoulderstand, or gentle neck rolls to relieve tension from being at your computer all day. Seek teachers or gurus who are true to their words, who honor yoga and the world with what they say *and* do. Sing. Pay a compliment. Tell a story. Tell a joke. Tell yourself the words you wait to hear from others. This, too, is yoga.

THROAT CHAKRA ESSENTIALS:

- Intention: I SPEAK
- Mantra: Ham
- Color: Blue
- Focus: Communication, clarity, expression.
- Asanas: Fish Pose, Shoulderstand, and gentle neck stretches like the ones shown.

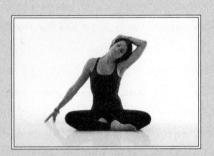

Neck Stretch 1
Gently drop your right ear toward your right shoulder
and lengthen your left fingertips away from your body. Next,
align your right forearm with the side of your face. Don't pull,
but let the weight of your arm help stretch your neck.

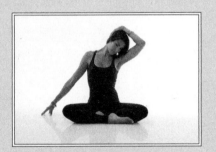

Neck Stretch 2
Now, tuck your chin in slightly and place your right palm
on the left side of your skull where it juts out (the occipital ridge).
Lightly press your head into your hand.

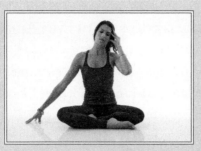

Neck Stretch 3
Finally, leave your head hanging down and use your right hand,
rather than your neck muscles, to lift your head.
Repeat on the left side.

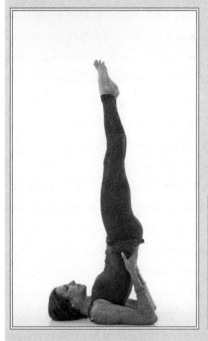

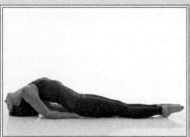

Shoulderstand

Matsyasana
(Fish)

Chakra 6: Third Eye | Ajna

The way I became friends with Olympic swimmer Kim Vandenberg, whom you'll meet later, is a fun story. It goes like this:

Kim: *Hi, my name is Kim.*

Me: *Hi, Kim. I'm Rebecca.*

And, now . . . we're friends.

It was intuitive and easy, the way kindred spirits recognize a similar spark or friends from a past life meet in this one. (I am a yoga teacher and can, therefore, say things like that without batting an eye.) In all seriousness, I know you've had similar experiences with some of the special people in your life. And you may have your sixth chakra to thank. Known as your ajna chakra, your third eye is located in your forehead. It governs aspects of life that your actual eyes cannot see. It's your sixth sense. Your intuition. It's what social scientist Malcolm Gladwell writes about in his bestselling book *Blink* as instinct. We all wish we had more of it, and the good news is that yoga can help strengthen your third-eye insight, just as it does your muscles.

Your eyes absorb raw information all the time. Your mind—and its years of accumulated wisdom and knowledge—guide how you respond to that information. Information is looking at the details of a résumé; wisdom is knowing whether your office culture will embrace the candidate. Information is player stats. Knowledge is the way a small player plays big or an emotional leader bonds a team. It's the eye through which my first yoga teacher saw me—not as an out-of-place sixteen-year-old but a glint of soul, like all the others, connected to all the others, exactly where she needed to be. The third eye senses opportunity and protects from danger. It reads people and situations beyond minute visual clues. It's the space, less furrowed than when we began, to which we connect our hands in prayer position and bow at the end of yoga class.

This energy point, like all the others we've discussed, is susceptible to getting blocked or clogged. At best, it's a smooth brow behind which lies superyogi X-ray vision powers of emotional intelligence. At worst, it's the spot you rub after staring at your computer all day or an exhausting meeting in which everyone talks in circles. Your brain is fried, vision blurry. You have a caffeine-withdrawal headache. You can't summon a creative thought to save your life. It's home to a thudding hangover, embedded in a permanent scowl, and ready for Botox.

"Your third eye needs a contact lens," quips the counter-culture yoga website Recovery Yogi, cofounded by my friend Joslyn Hamilton. The third-eye bon mot is the site's way of showing how important it is to trust our inner wisdom, rather than blindly following someone or something else. No matter where we are on the yoga path (or off of it), our intuition has important messages for us. We all experience times when our third eye does, indeed, need a contact lens of clarity. We're overcomplicating things that were once second nature. The job or relationship mojo is majorly lagging. The creative insight is kaput. When this happens, it's often better to stop forcing a solution or feigning insight we don't have. Rather, take a step back and try some activities that heighten intuition and rebalance the sixth chakra, including:

- *Meditation*: The section ahead shares plenty of helpful tips and styles of meditation. Try each of them until you find the one that helps you feel most steady, clear, and able to tap into your third eye insight.
- *A good night's sleep or* yoga nidra: Just a few nights of sleep deprivation can have devastating effects on your ability to connect with your intuition and think clearly. Get some rest, or try *yoga nidra,* a relaxing yoga style that evokes a sleeplike state.

- *Forehead massage*: place your hands in *anjali mudra* (prayer position). Bring your thumb knuckles to your third eye. Massage firmly but gently in circles, several times, both directions. Then, press your thumb tips into the inner corners of your eyes, just beneath the area where your brow bone juts out. Press inward and upward slightly. Not too hard. If you get the right spot, your whole face relaxes.
- *Acupuncture of this point.* It doesn't hurt, helps to relax the area, and, as my acupuncturist jokes, serves as a healthier alternative to injecting your face with poison. (Sorry gals, he means Botox.)
- *Creative visualization.* I recommend Shakti Gawain's books. Your subconscious doesn't know the difference between reality and a dream, so start visualizing your dreams, down to the smallest details of setting, sensations, even what you're wearing. When you practice your dreams inwardly, you strengthen your ability to manifest them outwardly (for a beginner visualization exercise, turn to page 199).

THIRD EYE CHAKRA ESSENTIALS:

- Intention: I SEE
- Mantra: Sham
- Color: Indigo
- Focus: Wisdom, clairvoyance, visualization.
- Asanas: Child's Pose

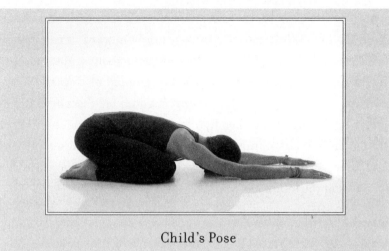

Child's Pose

Chakra 7: Crown | Sahasrara

Enlightened beings in history, such as Jesus, the Buddha, many of the gods and goddesses represented in the Hindu pantheon, and the gods of other ancient societies like the Egyptians, Greeks, and Romans are often depicted as radiating a coronal light, having a halo, or being encircled by a nimbus of energy around the top of their heads. As such, the crown chakra, located atop the head (where your soft spot was as a baby), is known as the physical home of your enlightenment. You could also visualize a cartoonish lightbulb that appears overhead when you have a really good idea. Whatever works for you. The sahasrara chakra represents the *aha* moments in life, when consciousness elevates to a higher level or you find a game-changing solution to a problem. A lightbulb goes on. Light is shed. Enlightenment found. You are plugged into something bigger and channeling its guidance.

The crown chakra is purple or white. It says "I understand." Its chant is *om* or the sound of silence. It loves Headstand, which offers fresh blood to your brain, and standing balances with an emphasis on the top of the head extending straight upward. It can delight in flashes of brilliance as much as doing the dishes. Your seventh chakra knows that the most important moment of your life is the one happening right now. Enlightenment does not discriminate. By activating the top of your head, uncapping your channel toward the Divine, the heavens, or higher understanding, or getting a good head scratch, we stimulate this pinnacle energy point. It's the culmination of all of the following.

- I am.
- I feel.
- I do.
- I love.
- I speak.
- I see.
- I understand.

When given the choice of a ponytail, pigtails, or barrettes, my friend's three-year-old daughter recently responded with her preference for the day, "My crown!" Wouldn't it be great if we could all do the same, activating our crown chakras at will, as if part of our outfits? Truthfully, we can. We have the capacity for greater understanding in each moment, beginning with—you guessed it—right now. It's a decision to look at any situation with new eyes, a willingness to see clearly, and a practice of being present to all the information around and wisdom within us. With this added knowledge about the energy patterns within the body, it's as though we're choosing what to wear for the day more enthusiastically and creatively. The only difference here is that your crown's sparkling brilliance is worn from the inside out.

CROWN CHAKRA EVERYDAY ESSENTIALS:

- Intention: I UNDERSTAND
- Mantra: Om
- Color: Purple/white
- Focus: Enlightenment, higher consciousness, and connection to spirituality.
- Asanas: Headstand and standing poses in which the crown is directed straight upward, such as Tree Pose.

The seven chakras in alignment make up a powerful energetic current within your body. Keeping this channel bright and balanced helps its internal glow radiate outward. This is an important job, which is why the five koshas are also here to help. The koshas encase and protect our inner light, giving us another way to acknowledge and delight in the practice of yoga and our experience of life.

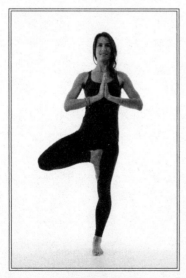

Vrksasana
(Tree Pose)

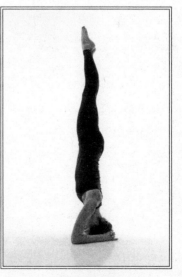

Sirsasana
(Headstand)

Chakra Essentials

Chakra name	*Location*	*Focus/Issues*	*Intention*
Muladhara/ root	Base of spine	Survival, security	I am.
Svadhisthana/ sacral	Lower back, belly, genitals, hips	Creativity, emotions, sexuality	I feel.
Manipura/solar plexus	Solar plexus	Willpower, courage	I do.
Anahata/heart	Heart, upper back, lungs, shoulders	Love, relationships	I love.
Vishuddha/ throat	Throat, neck	Communication, expression	I speak.
Ajna/third eye	Brow	Intuition, vision	I see.
Sahasrara/ crown	Top of head, cerbral cortex	Awareness, understanding, enlightenment	I understand.

Mantra	Color	Asanas	Other Healing Activities
Lam	Red	Standing and seated poses	Self-care for basic needs such as sleep, healthy food, and supportive people
Vam	Orange	Hip openers	Art and creative therapies
Ram	Yellow	Sun salutations, core work, and twists	Strong physical activities that evoke courage and accomplishment, such as hiking, surfing, or martial arts
Yam	Green	Backbends	Pranayama, listening to music, communing with nature
Ham	Blue	Postures that elongate/expose the neck	Singing, mantras (i.e. *japa* meditation)
Sham	Indigo	Child's pose	Visualization exercises, yoga nidra, massage, and acupuncture
Om	Purple/white	Inversions and standing balances	Meditation

CHAPTER 5

The Koshas:
Balancing the Layers of Your Being

Yoga tradition tells us that the body is comprised of five *koshas*, known as sheaths or layers. These layers represent the physical, energetic, mental/emotional, intellectual, and spiritual aspects of your body. Even the most linear-minded among you have probably experienced moments of kosha recognition—like when a colleague barges into your office before you've had coffee, and you say, "Whoa, whoa! Gimme a minute. I'm not here yet. . . . I mean, my body is here, but I'm not *here* yet." What you're saying is that your physical body might be at your desk, but your energetic body is back home in bed. Pretty soon you'll say, "My annamaya kosha is here, but my pranamaya kosha is still hitting the snooze button."

Or, maybe don't say that.

We intuit the body this way—that it's more than a physical structure of bones and muscles—but we forget because no one in the history of time ever approached you on a beach and said, "Damn, baby, your koshas look bangin' in that bikini." Yoga contends that the source of real beauty and balance begins inwardly and radiates outward, with the koshas protecting this inner light in successive layers like a hurricane lamp protecting its flame.

Or you can imagine koshas as a set of Russian nesting dolls. You can picture those, right? Think of the tiniest doll as the deepest core of your being, containing your chakra system, with all that energy and light zooming along your spine. When we care for and integrate each layer of our being, we feel balanced, clear, energized, steady, light, and peaceful. We are comfortable in our own skin. When one or more of the layers is neglected, we feel negatively affected. We are stressed, lethargic, frazzled, uninspired, or anxious. We might be beautiful or handsome on the outside but never truly feel that way on the inside. What I mean to say is that the first step to achieving some kind of imagined, perfect yoga body is realizing you already have it. You are it. The chakras capture and conduct your vitality up and down your body's central axis or spinal column. Meanwhile, the koshas protect this light and radiate it outward.

5 Steps to Nourishing Your Koshas

1. Embody how you want to feel.
2. Breathe as if it were the most important thing in your life. (It is.)
3. Master your emotions.
4. Beautify your brain.
5. Put some good in the world.

Physical Layer (Annamaya Kosha)

When you think about your body, you consider first your physical self—the outermost layer and what's known as the "food-apparent sheath." This is the annamaya kosha, which represents your body the way someone would describe you to police if you stole a case of kombucha from Whole Foods and ran. How tall you are; the color of your hair and skin; how you move (she hurdled the fire hydrant and took off down the alley); and how your bones, muscles, and flesh fit together to form your appearance. Most of all, it's also how you live in your own skin. Through this layer, you feel and filter the world. It's your most solid, tactile, external layer of being. It's dominated by the earth element and primarily derives sustenance from what you eat.

You make, create, and build things with this body. You dance. You hold hands. You feel this outermost layer when you jump in the ocean or make love. You celebrate it every time you break a healthy sweat or get caught in a downpour, turn your face to the sky, and laugh at how audacious Mother Nature can be. You indulge it with soft sweaters or fine thread counts. You protect it from too much sun exposure or sugar. The yoga practice that purifies and balances this layer of the body is *asana*—the physical postures performed in a yoga class.

There are also myriad life experiences that can be purifying to the physical layer of your body. These might include getting a massage, sitting in the steam room, or walking barefoot on a grassy lawn. Anything that is tactile, physically nourishing, or purifying counts. Most of all, we do our best to nourish our bodies with wholesome food, breaking bread with good people, and cooking for ourselves as often as we can because it's the healthiest thing you can do for your diet. You are what you eat, especially relative to this kosha. Because the stuff you feed your body *becomes* your "food body."

The body's health and fitness are paramount to how we do yoga and feel in our own skin, and we must never lose sight of the gift of our physicality as the vessel to express the rest of us. However, prioritizing the outermost layer while neglecting the others makes for a difficult relationship with our bodies. In the same way that physical attraction is important to a romantic relationship, but if there's no depth of respect or love beyond the superficial component, then the health of the whole bond deteriorates. Intellectually, we know this. We understand that we need our partners to value us beyond our looks. Why do we forget when it comes to ourselves, standing under the harsh lights of the dressing room? Why is body-snarking at others (whether celebrities in a magazine or people we actually know) or ourselves a thing?

Meanwhile, coveting the appearance of another person is like coveting anything else. You can let it illuminate what's important to you, transform it into useful action, or let it curdle into toxic jealousy. All of this can be part of yoga, a practice of elevating your awareness. The truth is that it's not the muscles or waistline you covet. Behind a longing for long legs or swooning for svelte shoulders is a desire for the feeling we think we'll achieve by having them. We want to feel something we see embodied in someone else.

What if ending your fat days or no longer feeling inferior on a mat next to someone more bendy or becoming than you were this simple: celebrate what your body *does* before how it *looks*. Never diminish others to feel better. Never diminish yourself. Take precious care of your outer layer. Move your body as much as you can. Sweat often. Eat well. Nourish yourself with good food and experiences. Stand confidently, even if you don't feel that way. As Buddhist monk and teacher Thich Nhat Hanh reminds us, "Sometimes, your joy is the source of your smile, but sometimes your smile can be the source of your joy." Remember what we learned about body language research: invoking a certain feeling physically can help inspire that feeling emotionally.

Prioritize sensation over appearance. How would you walk if you *felt* confident? Eyes downcast, fixated on your phone to avoid contact with anyone? Unlikely. How would you eat if you felt grateful for your physical health? Mindlessly, too fast, emotion stuffing, or guilt ridden? Nope. How would you practice yoga if you felt balanced and graceful? Would you hastily throw down your mat, snarl at the newcomer who sets up too close to you, and noisily leave before Savasana? Hardly.

Nourish yourself in every way. Experience the physical gifts of your life. Appreciate the aspect of yourself that comes in contact with all five elements: earth, water, air, fire, and space. Once you start recalibrating your brain to focus less on how individual parts of the body look, you'll get better at celebrating the way the whole functions. As a result, it will function better. It will start to shine, in fact.

Before you set another appearance-focused goal, chew on this thought again: *what do I want to embody?* What do your yoga or fitness aspirations embody? Grace, strength, speed, endurance, or indomitable will? Or, do you sense undercurrents of not good enough, not eating enough, and not vital enough? What fuels your yoga, workouts, and life? What nourishes you? Embody the real stuff. Crack the shell of the silly, self-consumed self. Toss the Photoshopped images. The best place for tabloids is the recycling bin. Ditch the diet soda. Feed yourself, and feel your *Self*. Make a bright, strong home in your own skin. Embody it. Embrace it. There is nothing more stunningly, honestly beautiful.

··

ANNAMAYA KOSHA QUESTIONS:

··

What do I want to embody?
What physical experiences nourish me?
When am I most comfortable in my skin?

··

Energetic Layer (Pranamaya Kosha)

In addition to your physical appearance, the energy you exude also characterizes who you are and contributes to how you feel in your body. It's the second layer of the subtle body, known as the pranamaya kosha. You can think of it as your energetic layer or "air-apparent sheath." You'll recognize the word *prana*, which means breath or life force, and has its own limb of yoga, which we discussed in Chapter 2. So, yes, when you're too busy to get to yoga class, sitting still and paying attention to your breath counts as practice. And those who quip that they're not flexible enough to do yoga will be happy to know that if you can breathe, you can do yoga.

If something has breath, it's alive. It's a *vital sign*. The more you focus on it, the more alive you become. Learn to control it, use its current wisely, and your whole being thrives. Your mind is calmer. Your thoughts are clearer, with edges sharpened and defined rather than tumbling into one another or pinging around too fast. Some may argue that focusing on your breath doesn't influence the look of your body, but I would place a handsome bet that someone who is in the moment, listening to his/her breath, does not emotionally eat a carton of ice cream. Are you starting to catch this yoga body drift? The physical layer relies on all the others. Health and beauty are multidimensional.

The yoga practice that directly influences the energetic layer of who you are is called *pranayama* (i.e., breathwork or breathing exercises). Perhaps you're already looking forward to trying a favorite from pages 53–56. Breath control is the quickest route to shifting energy, reviving inspiration, and reconnecting to a sense of self. The simple skill of paying attention to one, deep, conscious breath after another is grounding, healing, and even spiritual. You may recall that the translation of the Latin word *inspirare* is *to breathe spirit into*.

Befitting this connection, B.K.S. Iyengar describes prana as "God's breath," in his book *Light on Life*.

Breath is spiritual espresso. Starbucks coffee but better and cheaper. It perks us up, and instead of being on every street corner, it's available in every moment. We don't have to wait in line. What morning coffee is to bleary commuters, breath is to yoga. (To be candid, I don't drink coffee, but my morning tea ritual has the same effect.) Every inhalation is an invitation of new energy into our bodies and lives. We welcome in something we need, namely oxygen. However, we can also think of it as the breath of some specific energy we need: healing, creativity, or strength. Every exhalation is an opportunity to release old energy, as well as carbon dioxide. We let go of something we no longer need: stress, doubt, or fear. When you really think about it, a single breath is the beginning of everything you do in your lifetime, and attention to it places you in the moment of pure potential, the present. Just as oxygen is crucial for maintaining a fire, pranayama is the bellows for our inner flame. Take a breath, and your light brightens.

The air-apparent sheath or breath body influences the air in our lungs and around us, as each person emits energy simply by breathing and being. For instance, when you leave a room, taking air and energy with you, there is a feeling left behind, as was recounted in the earlier story I shared about His Holiness and JFK Jr. What is the feeling you leave behind? What would you like it to be? Do people feel more grounded, energized, or calm? The energetic layer of ourselves has the power to crack the toughest expressions, melt the chilliest of hearts, and ultimately let people know that everything will be OK, even in moments of crisis. *Oh, thank goodness, you're here.* Nobody's talking about how you look in that dress. They're talking about how you make them feel through the life force you exude.

If the first kosha represents a feeling of being at home in your own skin, think of your second kosha as the windows of this home, which let in fresh air, light, and your favorite sounds from outside—rain, birds, a foghorn at sea. When the energy in our houses, apartments, or dorm rooms feels stale or stagnant, we open a window. In our bodies, we take a giant, life-giving breath. Technically, we don't need to learn to breathe since we've done it our whole lives. It was the most important moment of our birth actually. Our mothers, fathers, the doctors, nurses, midwives, or doulas all waited for our first gasp of air, after exiting the womb, and the cry that followed. *I am here, World. I breathe your air.*

<hr>

Pranamaya Kosha Questions:

<hr>

What inspires me?

How do I want people to feel when I leave the room?

What unhealthy behavior or stuck energy do I want to change in myself? Before I engage in it, I will take five long, slow breaths (five-count inhale, five-count exhale). Repeat.

<hr>

Emotional Layer (Manomaya Kosha)

If a yoga class or pose has ever stirred strong emotion in you, whether love, loathing, or a puddle of tears (probably in Half Pigeon), then you intuitively understand the manomaya kosha, the mental or emotional layer of our being, characterized by the contents of our minds and how we feel about them, such as memories, fears, thoughts, likes, and dislikes. Since these things are impermanent (how many of us didn't like Brussels sprouts or beets as a child and could live on them now or previously hated a certain yoga pose and eventually grew to love it?), and yoga is about encompassing and unifying all the layers of our being, our job as yogis is to master our emotions so that they don't master us, on or off the mat. Through practices that steady emotions and our impulses in response to them, we learn to balance this layer of ourselves. It's important to feel our emotions as they are, yet remember that our emotions do not define us, and we don't want them to block our inner, unchanging, and Infinite light.

Practices to balance and burnish this kosha include meditation, bhakti (chanting), Karma yoga (acts of service to benefit others), and asana. Hip openers, for example, are notorious for unearthing stored emotions. Meanwhile, forward bends are among the most calming and cooling yoga poses we do. Backbends, on the other hand, are exhilarating, which is great when you need an energetic boost but might cause more disquiet if you're already prone to anxiety. We also each have strategies of our own that we know work for us. Perhaps you have a patch of sandy beach or quiet woods where your heart becomes still, a therapist's couch where you can talk freely, or the favorite kitchen table of a friend or family member where your body and soul are fed. To transcend your emotional layer, it helps to ask yourself a question I associate with this kosha.

How do you want to feel?

I pose this question to my students, and it's one I ask myself before beginning anything worth anything: taking a yoga class, running a race, starting a creative endeavor, you name it. How do you want to feel? I believe this type of awareness and intention is nothing short of life-changing because if you know how you want to feel, you can act accordingly. It helps to frame this question around something that is important to you, which you're about to undertake. If you know you want to feel relaxed after yoga, you can't peek at your cell phone during class (yes, we've seen you). If you want to feel joyful, you can't contort and compete with the yogi on the next mat over. If you want clarity, you must meditate. You have to make focusing on one breath at a time your first, second, third, and fourth priority. Your asana can come fifth. The music (if there is any) comes seventy-ninth. How do you want to feel when you walk out of the yoga studio . . . close the negotiation . . . finish the heart-to-heart conversation?

The more present you become to your manomaya kosha, the more honest you are with your emotions, the better you can master them. We recall Patanjali's original description of yoga's purpose as "stilling the fluctuations of the mind," so that we can be more present more often. On the other hand, ignore your emotions or impulsively respond to them all the time, and they will run the show.

Put simply, happiness is most available to people who are responsible for the contents of their consciousness. Take the inspiration of Nelson Mandela. While serving twenty-seven years in a South African prison for opposing apartheid, he drew solace and salvation from the poem "Invictus" by William Ernest Henley. Here's the poem's final verse:

> *It matters not how strait the gate.*
> *How charged with punishments the scroll.*
> *I am the master of my fate.*
> *I am the captain of my soul.*

The koshas take cues from each other and from the chakras as well, since this whole concept of the energetic anatomy works in concert: bundle by bundle of energy and layer by layer of being, all wrapped around our soul, Self, or atman. Like children or goldfish, each chakra and kosha requires care and balance. Feed them, but not too much. Be supportive, but don't hover or tap the glass. The emotional layer, in particular, can override the rest. Think of how the mother of a newborn might be physically depleted and exhausted, but her emotions are vibrating at such a high frequency that she experiences less fatigue. The emotions that accompany a feeling of immediate danger or deep romantic love are so intense that they can actually alter the chemicals in our bodies, specifically our hormones. We experience superhuman strength or speed as adrenaline courses through our bodies to protect us. After sex, we experience surges of oxytocin, dopamine, and prolactin, feel-good chemicals that make us amorous, happy, and cuddly.

Our emotions represent an element of our being that greatly influences all the others, from appearance to energy level. Depression makes people tired, for example. Anxiety makes it difficult to sit still or focus. Remember, we're working inward, toward the source of our energetic light. If one layer is clouded or neglected, the light is dimmer through our outermost layer. Our mental/emotional state of being influences how we carry our bodies, what we eat, how much or how well we sleep, our desire to exercise or lack thereof, and the habitual facial expressions we make (e.g., scowling, furrowing, laughing, smiling). When we feel gloomy, we're more likely to look that way. When we're aglow with passion or joy, there's a ripple effect through our whole being. Then, these emotions are further reinforced by the energy we attract with our scowling or smiling. I'm sure you can guess that each evokes more of the same. The key is to use our emotions to our advantage more often than our detriment through being present and practice.

manomaya kosha questions:

How do I want to feel?

Which people, places, and activities nurture and balance my
emotional life?

Describe what emotional balance feels like in your body—how do
you stand, sit, move, and breathe?

Intellectual Layer (Vijnanamaya Kosha)

If you've ever worked at a job that was no longer intellectually stimulating or taken a class you found so boring that it put you to sleep faster than spa music featuring ocean waves or rain forest sounds, you know what happens when the vijnanamaya kosha, your intellectual body, feels neglected. Think about your energy level in moments like these. When the wise and whip-smart layer of who you are, craving growth and learning, feels neglected and dusty, the rest of the body experiences low energy, lethargy, or a sensation of lemme-outta-here-I-can't-take-it-anymore. We want to crawl out of our skin or under our desks, hit the office vending machine hard at 3:00 p.m. (or 10:00 a.m. for that matter) in hopes that a sugar high can salvage an inspiration low, or flee to greener pastures, sandy beaches, anywhere but here.

Does this mean we need to quit the job or drop the class? Maybe. Maybe not. Sometimes we need the job or must fulfill the course requirement. But we also need to find intellectual stimulation somewhere and access our inner layer of wisdom. Otherwise, we may end up dozing through too much of life or hiding under our desks (metaphorically speaking) while more exciting and engaging experiences, opportunities, and people pass us by.

At a certain point, I got very tired of hearing well-meaning yogis, teachers in particular, say that *yoga is about much more than the poses* without any further explanation. Few yoga classes serve up this insight, and most of what I saw was a lot of fitness laced with pop psychology. In many cases, it seemed like once a student had a substantial grip on the asana practice and wanted to know more about the study, meaning, and wisdom of yoga, they had but one option at their disposal: fork over 3,000 dollars to their local studio and attend a yoga teacher–training program.

What if I don't want to teach yoga?

Doesn't matter. Teacher training is for anyone who wants to deepen his or her practice.

Can I deepen my practice without spending 3,000 dollars?

No.

I'm kidding, of course. However, this imagined dialogue wasn't far from the truth for a long time. Today, there are more options. Because, for as far as the yoga movement's pendulum had swung toward fitness, it's swinging back. Teachers are more educated. People genuinely want to know more about yoga's roots and applications off the mat. Meditation is accepted and endorsed by everyone from the medical community to pro athletes.

I started the Om Gal Book Club as a way to address the need to stretch and strengthen our brains as well as our bodies with the help of yoga. It's a small group of women, in my corner of the universe, who meet every other month. Coincidentally, the inspiration came from one of my private yoga students, a prominent and beloved philanthropist who has since passed away. One evening I showed up at her home to teach our regular yoga session and the expansive and elegant dining table was in a different location. "I hosted book club last night," she explained. We often talked about books to start or close our practice, and, over time, I realized how natural this combination was. My book club began soon thereafter with a desire to give people an opportunity to understand yoga in a deeper way, explore its greater themes, and talk about how these themes emerged in the books we'd read and lives we live. It was a way for yogis to beautify their brains, not just focus on the work of the body. And it's free. To date, the currency exchanged is a communal and intellectual kind, and it's a personal bow to my former student's generous spirit. Much is made in the yoga community about listening to your body, and this is invaluable advice. However, we also need to listen to the hum and pulse of our intellectual layer, comprised in part by the one hundred billion neurons in our happily firing brains, which create synapses, and, according to renowned neurologist V.S. Ramachandran, form everything that we are, including our ambitions, passions, and even our private sense of self.

Early in my career as a yoga teacher, I worked as the lead teacher at the Baptiste Power Yoga Institute in Boston. Hot yoga was, well, *hot*, and I was simultaneously the youngest and most experienced teacher at the busiest yoga studio in the world, at that time. But let me be candid about what this hot job actually entailed: I taught roughly fifteen ninety-minute classes per week, in a room heated to around one hundred degrees. This schedule generated so much sweat-drenched laundry that I could barely keep atop it before needing to buy more (expensive) yoga clothing. No weekends. No vacation time, sick time, or 401(k). My body ached. My vocal cords strained. I wearied of teaching the same thing over and over again, and the following occurred: my brain melted. Maybe it was the temperature. Maybe it was the lack of intellectual stimulation. Probably it was both. But, that's what it felt like. It was serious burnout, and I needed a change.

I left the yoga scene and went to work for a magazine. I wore shoes at work again, and it felt wonderful. I started a blog, where I could give voice to the aspects of yoga that always fascinated my mind and fired up my spirit. I scaled back my teaching almost entirely, only to ramp it up again later. When something is your *dharma* (your sacred calling), you don't choose it. It chooses you.

The vijnanamaya kosha helps us make choices like these. It decides, discerns, studies, and scrutinizes. Whereas the mental/emotional body that precedes it represents our incessant thoughts and feelings, the intellectual body is characterized by discernment and reason. It's the part of you that bought this book. It's the layer of your being, which, while in a yoga pose, understands not just a pose's mechanics but also its consciousness. This layer likes making connections, the practice of yoga to its greater philosophy and ways in which it might help some people answer the larger questions we all ponder, like who am I and what is my purpose.

··

VIJnanamaya kosha questions:

··

Who am I?_____

What is my purpose? _____

When does my intellectual layer thrive? _____

··

Blissful Layer (Anandamaya Kosha)

The word *ananda* means bliss, which brings us to the body's final layer, known as the anandamaya kosha. It's the spiritual, most inner layer of your being, and closest to your deepest self (*atman*). I think of it as the way people sparkle when they're doing things they love or are in love, when we're aligned with our soul's desire. It's our own personal supply of phosphorescence, inwardly located but outwardly visible. It's also the part of us that is connected to everyone and everything else in the universe.

When mythology scholar Joseph Campbell famously wrote, "Follow your bliss," he was talking about the path each of us walks as the hero of our own tale. He noticed and outlined reoccurring archetypes for heroes throughout time and across cultures in his book *The Hero with a Thousand Faces*, among others. In a similar (albeit subtler) way, the koshas map our yoga journey. We experience the poses physically. We add our breath, and by doing so, we synergize mind and body. We're more aware of our body's vital energy. We experience mental and emotional shifts. We learn to watch our thoughts, harness the power of our minds, and anchor our emotions. Then, we use our intellectual body to consider the whole experience of yoga more fully. We discern how we will practice as well as live. Finally, we might feel a state of bliss, something we've possessed all along and only needed to remember and return to.

People who are in touch with their bliss sparkle with energy. They are interested in life and interesting to be around. They're not schlepping through one life with another unfulfilled one inside them, nor are they unaware of how extraordinary an ordinary existence can be. There are several ways to access and purify your blissful body. Some of these include devotional practices such as prayer, music, or anything that connects you to your experience of a higher power and the totality of the universe. Most of all, it's about being convinced of our own inherent goodness and seeing this possibility for goodness, heroism even, in everyone else on our path.

Derek Beres is a music producer and yoga teacher in Los Angeles who uses music in a very skilled manner to summon the spiritual side of his students. Instead of aiming to entertain or distract students with a cool playlist, he trains ears and hearts to feel the music and use it to anchor their physical (*asana*), contemplative (*dharana*), and meditation (*dhyana*) practices. One of the ways he does this is through an exercise he developed called "song tasting." Like wine tasting, the objective is not to chug a glass to get drunk, it's to taste a small pour to pick up the subtle qualities of the varietal. Only instead of sensing tannins and top notes, yogis identify emotions conveyed through music. What is the song about? What is it trying to convey? Which part of the human condition is moved? Beres describes this skill set as a way to build emotional intelligence and empathy. Students are asked to close their eyes and sit comfortably, in meditation or a favorite restorative yoga posture.

Thirty seconds of music is played, and then, the yogis are asked what they heard and felt.

The first song I heard in one of Derek's tastings sounded triumphant and expansive to me. I saw Native American warriors on horseback or herds of buffalo galloping across the plains. It sounded like a song for exploration or battle. When I shared my answer with the group, Derek laughed a little. Maybe the buffalo comment was a little much?

Nope.

Derek was laughing at the accuracy. The song was by a band from the Tuva Republic that herds wild reindeer. How on earth did I know that? I laughed, too. Of course I didn't *know* it; I felt it. I listened with my spirit as well as with my ears. So did the rest of the class. When he played a song invoking sadness, the response was poignant. Some people were moved to tears. Sad music often occurs through minor keys, we learned. Coincidentally, music composed in minor keys has been the most popular on the Billboard charts since the late sixties.

There's that signature quote by Pierre Teilhard de Chardin, "We are not human beings having a spiritual experience; we are spiritual beings having a human experience," and this exercise felt like a small way to remember what that big feeling is like. Anytime you tap into something bigger than yourself, even for thirty seconds, when something touches your heart deeply, maybe breaks it a little, or hoists it straight up into the air, like a ballerina lifted by her partner, your blissful layer becomes more pure and clear. When you become more empathetic, feel reassured of the universe's loving nature, the connection of all beings, the presence of God, or your highest self, you know you've traveled through all the layers of your being. This is not a workout per se. It's the working inward of your now-balanced yoga body, anchored by a beautiful mind and strong spirit. We won't be blissful all the time, but through our own take on yoga practice and care for the yoga body as a whole, we're never too far away.

Finally, when we do wander from our own inner brightness, the return can often be kick-started by the simplest expression of our highest self: an act of spiritual generosity toward someone else. By now, you probably should have figured out that this yoga body program wouldn't include weight lifting but, rather, spirit lifting instead. Because nothing makes us feel lighter than putting some goodness in the world.

ANANDAMAYA KOSHA QUESTIONS:

How am I the hero of my own journey?

How am I following my bliss?

What is one act of spiritual generosity, small or large, that I can do for someone else?

Now, how will I put it into action?

Om Expert:

Derek Beres, yoga teacher, music producer, author, and secular Buddhist.

His Om Thing:

Merging music and neuroscience to strengthen one's emotional response.

What he says:

There's only one place in the world that music happens: inside of our heads. Nothing affects so many regions of our brains at once as music. Strangely it is the only nonessential activity (from an evolutionary perspective) that people across the planet partake in. We take immense pleasure in listening to and performing music, and have created a wide range of sounds to mimic our emotions: the sweeping sadness of the cello, the glorious victory of violins, the triumphant battle march of trumpets and percussion. While cultures are in part defined by their music, we can also utilize it for our own personal mental and emotional development. While the term "spiritual" is employed in a variety of ways, I can think of nothing deeper than being able to control (and not be controlled by) your emotions. We know, in large part thanks to the work of Richard J. Davidson, that meditation helps us create space in our brains by lengthening the time between an action happening and our response to that event. This means that meditation helps us not to be so reactive, using our emotions for our highest good instead of feeling used by them. Knowing that music also offers wonderful mental benefits, I co-created Flow Play, a yoga, music, and neuroscience program to help people understand the transformative power of meditating to music. Below is one meditation designed to help someone deal with anger. In it you will be asked to find a song with an Indian sitar, preferably during the alap (instrumental section with no percussion). Research conducted at the University of Berlin found that sitar music lowers levels of cortisol in the listener's blood. This meditation is useful even when you're not angry, and as Davidson's research has shown, it could help you cool off more quickly when faced with a challenging situation.

How You Can Do It:

- Find a slow, sitar-based song with no percussion. A few great examples: "Samadhi" by Shaman's Dream, "Meeting of Two Oceans" by Chinmaya Dunster.
- Hit play and take a comfortable seat; you can even lie down, as long as your spine is straight.
- Close your eyes and pay attention to the music. If your mind starts to wander to other thoughts, simply notice where it travels. Do your best to not create more stories out of the thoughts that arise. Instead, guide your attention back to the music.
- Notice the feelings inside of your body as the song progresses. Over time, the focus shifts to the feelings, as all emotions are first felt and then thought about. Try to keep your attention on the feeling of the song inside of you.
- Practice this for five to ten minutes each day. Recent research has shown that meditating for just five minutes a day for five weeks helped people deal with their emotions more effectively.
- Try to change the music at least once a week, if not more often. Once we learn a song, we begin to anticipate what's coming next, and this could be a distraction to simply being present with the song as it plays.
- Most important, enjoy! If meditation feels like work, you won't want to return to it. Even if you can only get to two or three minutes at first, stop while you're ahead. Over time you'll find that you crave longer durations.

....

I know many yoga books offer more finite prescriptions for feeling and looking your best. But in my opinion, the only way to feel beautiful, brawny, or happy in your own skin is to work in as well as work out. The only way to lose weight is to become more conscious about how you nourish and move your body, on every layer. If it's commonly accepted that people emotionally eat, doesn't it make sense that we could emotionally nourish ourselves to produce an opposite, more desirable effect? Physical and emotional health and strength begins with awareness, because the way you inhabit your inner environment reflects outwardly. We've always known that yoga supports our physical goals, but, if you're reading this book, you're ready to take it to the next level. You do yoga; therefore, you have a yoga body. Now you know what you want to embody. And anytime you forget, the yoga tools here will help you remember.

Part Three

The Mind

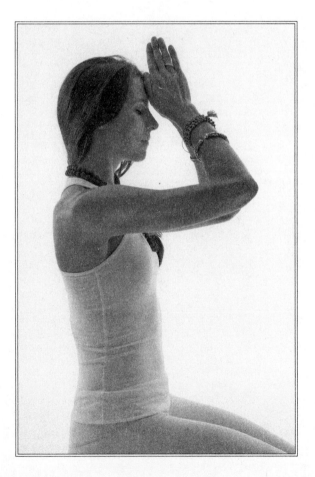

CHAPTER 6

Why Meditate?

As I was in the process of writing this book, my mornings started early. Many times by sunrise I was riding my bike across the Mass Ave. Bridge, over the Charles River, to a meditation center in Cambridge. Some days the sight of the Harvard crew boats gliding beneath the bridge, epitomizing efficiency and teamwork, as the sun rose above the gilded dome of the State House took my breath away. Ditto the air on frigid winter mornings when breathing through a thick scarf, wrapped ninja style around my face and helmet, still wasn't enough to ease the sting of the cold entering my lungs.

The meditation center is set back slightly from a busy street and protected by a fence. On the fence's gate is a small sign that reads: *Please Leave Open*. This refers to the gate. However, it could just as easily refer to the hearts and minds of the people who enter. The most common misconception about meditation is that the goal is to shut the gate of our mind on all thoughts, emotions, sounds, and distractions. Not only is this unrealistic, it's impossible. Knowing that we are thinking is a thought itself. And particularly when it comes to unpleasant thoughts or situations in life, it's not useful to numb ourselves into a zombie-like state. Instead, the goal of meditation is to observe our thoughts from a more conscious and centered place. We leave the gate open and, with practice, become more compassionate and discerning about what comes and goes. Most of us are highly conscious about the content stored in our smartphones, the content of our bank accounts, and the content of our closets, for example. Wouldn't it make sense to be equally, if not more, concerned with the contents of our minds—the originators of the whole experience of our lives?

As we've discussed with regard to the eight limbs, meditation precedes the ultimate goal of yoga: enlightenment, known as *samadhi*. In other words, meditation is the precursor to being fully awakened. For now, though, let's put the lofty goal of enlightenment aside and simply focus on leaving our hearts and minds open. Because, if having flexible hamstrings feels nice, having a flexible mind feels even better. Put another way, how we open and inhabit our minds influences every moment of our lives. Even if you're an exceedingly dedicated über yogi, reporting to your mat each day, you might spend somewhere between seven and fourteen hours a week on your mat. Yet, we live in our heads every minute, of every hour, of every day. By contrast, that's closer to 170 hours a week spent in your mind—where your hamstrings, booty, and biceps wield little influence. As you sleep, too, your subconscious mind is at work. Therefore, yoga's goal is to make this internal environment a hospitable one.

If your mind is as serene as an oasis in the Maldives, then you don't need yoga or meditation. But if your mind tends toward the partly cloudy, occasionally stormy, or potentially volcanic, you have the ideal conditions to practice mindfulness and create a more peaceful existence. As my favorite meditation teacher, Jon Kabat-Zinn, says, "Mindfulness cultivates an intimacy with a capacity we already have." We awaken to our own potential and the conscious choice we have of how we will show up in a given moment. Yoga practice is one doorway to mindfulness, to a layer of depth and capacity waiting within you, a serene destination requiring no travel.

Meditation is central to the ancient tradition of yoga but, more important, it's key to the lifestyle of a modern yogi. The Internet is, of course, among the greatest innovations in the history of humanity; it has changed, and often enhanced, the way we live, work, date, communicate, and even think. As we all know, this added bandwidth also comes with responsibility. If we aren't careful, we can become disconnected from what is actually happening in our lives at any given moment. We can avoid our feelings by zoning out, passing time, surfing, scrolling, and clicking. We can become so wired that we live our lives through our devices more than our hearts and minds. We can be incessantly connected to Friends and Followers and still feel disconnected from ourselves and lonely for true companionship. Enter the timeless and invaluable analog practice of meditation.

Ironically, at a time when more Americans than ever before are doing yoga, we are less present than we've ever been. We know we're more wired. But studies also show we are the most sleep-deprived, in-debt, addicted, obese, and medicated adult generation in history. To me, that data suggests that we need to improve our understanding and practice of yoga so that we can build happier and healthier versions of ourselves and our communities. We need to open the gate of the mind to the here and now and leave it open. Whatever enters and whatever life brings, we have a choice and capacity for how to handle it.

This section of the book is focused on the mind, which means that we will spend most of our time exploring meditation. This practice is yoga's most valuable tool for cultivating a mental state that is less distracted, more present, and more connected. Meditation helps you understand and, by extension, become more of yourself. It's also the polar opposite of common self-soothing behaviors like shopping, eating, or imbibing—actions that numb our senses, taking us out of the moment and away from ourselves. This isn't to say that going shopping or grabbing a glass of wine after a tough day is bad or unyogic behavior. Not at all. We're simply trying to be more aware of our choices and the intentions behind them. At its most basic level, yoga is an awareness practice, including when, where, and to what degree we avoid the present moment. Then, we practice gently returning to that moment, which, as I've said earlier, is the only one that's truly real: not a memory of the past or a guess at the future.

By developing skills of awareness and mindfulness, we enhance our capacity for life and even positively alter the structure of our brains, specifically in regions associated with memory, sense of self, empathy, and stress. In a 2011 study at Massachusetts General Hospital, researchers were able to demonstrate via magnetic resonance imaging (MRI) measurable changes in the brains of people who meditated for eight weeks versus a control group. These changes included marked increases in gray-matter density in the hippocampus, the region of the brain responsible for learning and memory, and in structures associated with self-awareness, compassion, and introspection, as well as decreased gray-matter density in the amygdala, which is connected to stress and anxiety. By becoming more present through meditation, your brain undisputedly gets stronger. You become better at making decisions, regulating your emotions, and experiencing less anxiety about life. Yes, just by breathing and sitting still for a few minutes a day. How cool is that?

If you've tried to meditate in the past but discovered it was hard, you are alone. I'm kidding! Meditation is difficult for ALL of us. It may be simple . . . Step one: sit still. Step two: breathe. Step three: repeat. But it has its challenges for everyone. I promise it gets easier, and as you're already beginning to see, the payoff is well worth it, for the reasons I've mentioned and many more.

Like much of modern life (and, often, yoga), we tend to assess worthiness by performance and outcome. This misconception is what makes meditation difficult. We think we're doing it wrong because we ascribe values of performance to it. We sit still for a few minutes, watch our minds race and churn, and think we've failed already. We grow frustrated that we can't stop the thinking mind. But here's the thing: the thinking mind *can't be stopped*, and meditation is not a performance-based activity. Unless there is someone out there who is better than you at being *you*? Didn't think so. . . . The best thing you can do for yourself as you venture into mindfulness or rejuvenate a lapsed meditation practice is to let go of what you believe meditation *should* be and, instead, experience yourself where you are, as you are. This shift not only makes meditation easier but also creates a sense of ease within us that stretches into all other aspects of life over time. Too often, yogis assume that meditation should feel as easy as it looks in pictures. It should feel like a mental ascension to a Buddhist monastery, on a mountaintop. It should be graceful, beautiful, and blissful. Brows do not furrow. Jaws do not clench. Noses do not itch.

The most liberating realization that I can offer is that this is precisely how meditation feels sometimes, and this isn't bad news. The nature of the mind is to wander, itch, and attach to expectations. This isn't a bad thing or a good thing; it's a just a thing. It just is. You're not doing it wrong, and you are not any less of a yogi than anyone else. Return to step one: sit still; step two: breathe; and step three: repeat. The only way to meditate badly is not to meditate at all. And the more you do it, the less dominance the difficult, boring, and itchy thoughts have over you. The purpose is not to be like a monk on a mountaintop, it's to spend time with the true nature of your own mind. Because the quality and direction of your attention is the greatest determinant of the quality of your life.

CHAPTER 7

How to Meditate: Five Essential Elements

J ust as there are countless styles of yoga, there are many ways to meditate, and, beyond meditation, an infinite number of other activities that can help to cultivate mindfulness. The key is finding what works for you. Some meditation styles are associated with spiritual paths (e.g., Buddhism). Others are secular, and this is what is meant by *mindfulness*. It is the style of meditation on which this book largely focuses. No matter how you choose to meditate, each style is built on the same basic principles.

Find a comfortable seat.

It can be intimidating to try to mimic those pictures of yogis meditating in full lotus position, only to feel massively uncomfortable within minutes if not seconds. I would strongly encourage you to view any meditation photos (including the ones in this book) with a grain of salt. I can tell you that while I felt relaxed and comfortable in my photo shoot, I was also listening to someone just outside the frame saying *add a hint of a smile* and *drop your chin slightly*. There was someone present to catch every flyaway hair and accidental scowl. As far as I can tell, you can't photograph inner peace. There are only photos that we might turn to as inspiration to help us achieve it.

The reality is that sitting still can be uncomfortable, but rather than assume we must be doing it wrong or it is dumb and foot numbing, we need to experiment with our preferred meditation position.

Some common favorites include Sukhasana (Easy Pose/sitting cross-legged), Padmasana (Full or Half Lotus), or Virasana (Hero Pose), all with the option of sitting on a meditation cushion (*zafu*), yoga block, or bolster. It's also perfectly OK to sit in a chair or lie down (as long as you will not fall asleep). If you tend to doze off during meditation, there's an important reason why: you need more sleep.

Sit tall.

Posture powerfully conveys body language and intention, inwardly and outwardly. You'll recall Amy Cuddy's research mentioned in Chapter 4 about how the act of changing our body position to a more open or confident stance, particularly with the chin slightly lifted to present a lengthened neck and throat, triggers the release of testosterone in both men and women and makes us *feel* more confident. Jon Kabat-Zinn recommends sitting in a posture that reflects *dignity*. This characteristic stands, err, sits in contrast to passively slumping or rigidly overexerting. "Everybody seems to instantly know that inner feeling of dignity and how to embody it," Kabat-Zinn writes in his go-to meditation guide *Wherever You Go There You Are*. I would add that you'll want to pay particular attention to your heart and shoulders (think: fourth chakra) by opening your chest and relaxing your shoulders.

Remain still.

Remember: your nose will itch. Your foot will tingle. The phone will ring. A child will interrupt and wonder what's for breakfast. As best as you can, let these experiences arise and dissipate. If you need to scratch your nose lightly, change the position of your foot, or mindfully answer your child, that's OK. There are no rules for what makes a good meditation, no point deductions for nose itches. You're cultivating the skill of being more present in your life—not ignoring your children. However, the mind seeks and overindulges in distractions, especially for beginner meditators. Your goal is to maintain stillness, with minimal adjusting, fidgeting, or breaking focus. Make an adjustment if necessary, but give it no more energy or momentum than needed. Over time, the distractions will lessen or, more accurately, your relationship and reactivity to them will change. On the morning I wrote this chapter, for example, I meditated to the sound of garbage trucks creating a ruckus in the alley behind my apartment. I watched my thoughts get sidetracked into an idealized world where garbage trucks weren't so inconsiderate of my yoga needs. Then, I realized how apropos it was: the trucks take my trash, and meditation clears my junk thoughts.

Start small.

Similar to rewiring the mind and body for any health habit, such as getting more exercise or eating better, it's best to make small changes and build incrementally. Just as you wouldn't attempt Bird of Paradise Pose (a tricky arm bind combined with balancing on one leg) before first learning to bind your arms, you probably shouldn't sign up for a two-week silent Vipassana retreat before trying ten minutes at home. Life transformation starts with small and sustainable changes. If meditation is exceedingly hard for you, try just five minutes per day. Setting a timer is crucial (an iPhone with the harp ring tone works well) because it ensures you won't be distracted by watching the clock.

It's not easy, but if we can't stand to be with ourselves for five uninter-rupted minutes now, how can we expect to get along with ourselves for a lifetime? This small start—these five minutes of being present, on purpose, without judgment*—is a game-changer.

Stop waiting for the perfect conditions.

I'm suspicious of anything that proclaims, feigns, or status up-dates perfection. It's usually inauthentic, inaccessible, or painfully boring. Not to mention that waiting for the perfect conditions or the "right time" is the best way to ensure you never do anything. You don't need the perfect meditation cushion, candle, outfit, mantra, space in your home, or teacher to meditate. You just need to start.

And while you're at it, throw out the perfect life plan in which a relationship, job, marriage, or family happen according to a sched-ule. You're not a train. You're a person, with a soul. Sit quietly for a moment and listen to it. Relieve yourself of the belief that you will be content when you have accumulated perfect houses, lawns, dogs, or children on holiday cards. The conditions you need to be happy are not outside you. They are contained within you: right here, right now. There's nothing to change but your mind, and there's no need to wait a moment longer to be the person you want to be. "The only Zen found on tops of mountains is the Zen you bring there," author of *Zen and the Art of Motorcycle Maintenance* Robert Pirsig wrote. The same could be said for your meditation cushion.

Helpful Tools

So far, we've established that meditation is challenging but worth-while, which should not come as a surprise since anything re-

....

* The definition of mindfulness is from Jon Kabat-Zinn; see Bibliography.

warding is challenging. There are also some basic tools, which you already possess, to make meditation easier. If asanas are the way for yogis to train the body to be flexible, strong, and balanced, meditation is the mind's training program for cultivating the same qualities. Like determining which yoga practice is best for you, you need to find your favorite way to meditate as well. Once you've found your preferred seat, you'll need to tinker with the tools below to find your ideal meditation mojo. Bear in mind, each style utilizes or prioritizes these tools differently. Your om thing begins and ends with you, so try what sounds appealing, evaluate what feels right, and refine the practice that encourages the most awareness and inner quiet for you.

Prana

As we know, the quickest way to shift or uplift our energy isn't delivered via a jolt of caffeine but through taking a deep breath. When you focus on a single breath, you place yourself in the present moment, since it is physically impossible to take a breath in the future or the past. Therefore, whenever you pay close attention to a single breath, you are practicing being fully present. If you find your mind agitated or bored in meditation, return to the sensation of one breath at a time. You don't need to manipulate the breath in any way. This isn't pranayama. It's merely awareness of your breath and life force itself. From here, the present, all things are possible.

Drishti

To increase our focus and sense of peace, we must consciously decrease the stimulus entering our eyes and ears from outside sources. Just like the Dalai Lama recommended. For meditation purposes, this means that the quieter the environment, the better. We also need to direct our *drishti* or gaze to one specific visual landmark. If your eyes wander, so will the mind. Common drishtis for meditation include downcast and gentle eyes (on the floor, for example) or closed eyes. When eyes are closed, they can still maintain a drishti. To do this, try looking toward the inside of your forehead (i.e., third eye/sixth chakra), into your heart, or toward the earth in front of you. Giving your eyes direction directs your mind, and directing your mind determines the focus of your life. As you aim to improve the quality of your attention, consider the quality of your gaze as an important stepping-stone. How do you look upon the world, yourself, and others?

Mantras

Thoughts are the food of our minds, each containing varying nutrition levels. Some thoughts, perhaps passionate ones summoned by great literature or true love, for example, energize us. They're like organic vegetables from the local farmers' market. Other thoughts, like those associated with jealousy or gossip, deplete us. They're like Cheetos with their artificial everything: flavor, color, smell. They're not real. They don't nourish the body or serve it in any way, and we're better off without them. A mantra is a nutrient-dense thought, one that feeds your best self and intentions. The translation of mantra actually means "mind protecting," and it refers to a sacred word or phrase repeated to aid concentration in meditation. Mantras help anchor the mind, build mental discipline, and wire healthy thought patterns into the mind's deepest layers.

As mentioned previously, unhealthy thought patterns (*samskaras*) include the negative or damaging things we think, say, and do, often reflexively. Over time, these thoughts create deeply in-layed grooves in our brains; the more we repeat a certain behavior, the more the brain becomes hardwired to respond in the same way. Soon we may find ourselves in the throes of unhealthy habits and behavior patterns, anything from negative self-talk to numbing with food or substances to choosing the wrong romantic partners, over and over again. When you consider all the aimless or toxic thoughts we habitually think—like junk food with its empty calories—it becomes clear that focusing the mind through meditation is as healthful to the mind as giving up junk food is for our bodies. The best way to avoid or put an end to unhealthy habits is to change the relationship you have to them in your mind. Quick aside: the best beauty secret in the world by far and away is get your mind right.

The most important aspect of a mantra is not its actual meaning. Instead, it's the reaction or thought vibration evoked within the yogi when it is repeated. With enough repetition, we implant a powerful and intentional secret weapon in our minds, like a song lyric from high school wired so deeply that we never forget it. Wouldn't it be better if you could be more in control of which thought soundtrack played most often in your mind? This is the power of mantras. *Om* is the most popular mantra in yoga, and you can always start there. Next, try Sanskrit words or English words that resonate with you. You will know them as soon as you hear or speak them because they vibrate at the frequency of your highest self. Mantra meditation is known as *japa*, which you'll learn more about later, along with some favorite mantras to try.

Mudras

Used in yoga and meditation, a *mudra* is a hand gesture; however, it technically translates to mean a *seal*—as in, sealing a letter. Applied in this way, hand positions connote specific intentions for meditation. They serve as body language you send yourself and seal into your being. On hectic days, when life feels shaky and unsure, you need the grounding sensation of bhu mudra. When your heart is heavy, you need padma mudra, which evokes sensations of openness and warmth in the heart chakra. Mudras are among my favorite tools to help focus the mind and prepare for meditation. To evoke any of the following intentions, try one of these mudras on your own for five to ten deep breaths.

To ground: Bhu mudra

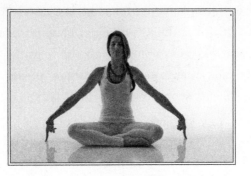

To offer peace or gratitude: Anjali mudra

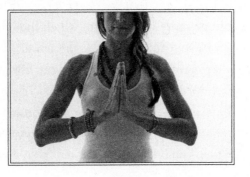

To evoke love and heart healing: Padma mudra

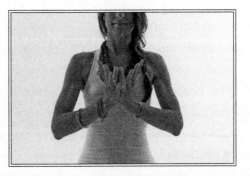

To remove obstacles: Ganesha mudra. Create an "obstacle" by hooking your hands as shown. Inhaling, tense your muscles and pull strongly in opposite directions. Exhaling, relax. Repeat six times, then switch your grip and repeat on the other side. Finally, place your hands over your heart, one atop the other. Breathe and listen inward.

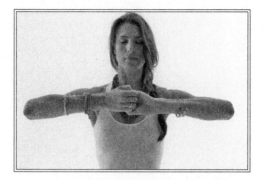

To symbolize connection (to yourself, others, the wisdom and tradition of yogis who came before you): Jnana mudra

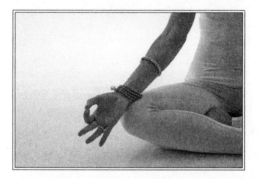

To hold space: Dhyani mudra

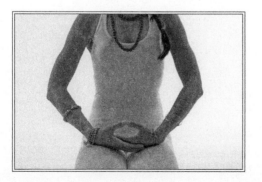

CHAPTER 8

Make It Your Om:
Finding Your Meditation Style

The value of meditation is not in its performance or execution but in its process and the space it creates in our minds. It nurtures our being, as if a direct response to the incessant *doing* of our modern lives. Without learning to *be*, we otherwise risk frittering away life and brainpower with too much busyness and not enough stillness, too much grasping and not enough gratitude, too much mental clutter and not enough space.

The irony is that the quicker life moves and the greater our need to slow down, the more we tend to speed up. Those of you with children are familiar with this behavior. Just before naptime, toddlers move exponentially faster when they need a nap—sometimes to the point of becoming clumsy and tripping over their own tiny feet as the fatigue sets in and coordination short-circuits. I experienced this with my own goddaughter, Adrianna. It didn't take long for me to realize that I wasn't doing her any favors by delaying her naps in favor of more playtime . . . and then to see that most of us do the same thing.

When we feel overwhelmed, overworked, overscheduled, or overly emotional, we rarely have the clarity to do less, slow down, and sit still, if only for a few minutes. It might be physical, emotional, or spiritual fatigue, but the alternative eventually leads to a wipeout. When we don't take the time to reset and recharge, we're more likely to lash out, emotionally eat, sabotage the relationship, fall ill from the stress, or spend money, as if inner peace were something one could buy. The daunting news is that the price we pay for not being present is a steep one when compounded over a lifetime, taking a physical and emotional toll that can lead to stress, anxiety, depression, and the sinking suspicion that you deserve better. YOU DO. The good news is that each of us has the power to address and remedy the spiritual burnout we all experience from time to time.

Here are some ways of meditating to clear the mind, calm the body, and recharge the spirit:

Awareness

Awareness meditation (sometimes referred to interchangeably as mindfulness meditation) is the simplest kind. Follow the five essential elements first introduced in Chapter 7: find a comfortable seat, sit tall, remain still, start small (set a timer), and let go of needing the perfect conditions. Any time you catch yourself lost in thought, identify it as *thinking* and return to the experience and skill of focusing on the present moment. Breathe naturally, and use the sensation of your breath in your nose, throat, and lungs to ground and focus you. If you're struggling, you can also try counting one breath at a time. Note that while it's important to build a strong and flexible mind through regular meditation, you can also use these skills throughout your day, just as you stitch together short exercise sessions by forgoing the escalator for the stairs or biking to work. It's not a separate, concentrated workout, but it creates a foundation for the health of your body. Similarly, you can do awareness meditation in pockets of time throughout your day: on a crowded subway, in the waiting room at the doctor's office, or—my favorite—during an emergency root canal before I left to teach a yoga retreat in Mexico. I could have chanced scheduling the procedure for when I had more time and felt more prepared after the trip. But, like a wise guru in a white coat, my dentist illuminated reality, "Sure, you can chance it. You might be okay till after you return, or the tooth might turn on you a few days from now, while you're in Mexico. The fact is: it's not going to get any better, and the time is now." He was right. It wasn't fun, but it was the right thing to do. I learned a valuable lesson that day: always start with the reality of now (and have a great dentist). I also realized how essential meditation has become to my ability to face daily challenges—like making an unexpected and important decision with a clear head, managing physical discomfort, and soothing anxiety. Ironically, my first yoga teacher, in the converted firehouse on Cape Cod, was fond of saying that any yogi could meditate in a dark room lit with candles and incense. But could you meditate at the dentist? Thank goodness I paid attention.

Japa

Japa meditation prioritizes the use of mantra, a mind-protecting and anchoring utterance repeated aloud or silently to oneself. Often, yogis use mala beads on which to count the number of repetitions of their mantras, much like rosary beads. Typically, malas contain 108 beads. This number is significant for many reasons, which we'll discuss in Chapter 10. You may feel inspired to maintain that tradition or use a multiple of 108. The reality of being a modern yogi is that you may not have time for 108. So, perhaps try 54, 27, or 9. What you say is up to you, and it will change depending on your physical, mental, and spiritual needs. Here are some staple, traditional Sanskrit mantras that might work for you:

Om:

The sound of the Universe, Universal Consciousness, Oneness, and connection to the Infinite. Simple and straightforward, a heartfelt om vibrates at a powerful frequency. More than hearing it, you feel it. You feel connected, whole, and alive.

Om shanti:

The word *shanti* means peace. This is a wish of peace for all.

Om namah shivaya:

We'll discuss the gods and goddesses who appear regularly in modern yoga, such as Shiva, in Chapter 10. As a head start, this mantra nods to Shiva, the god of destruction and creation, therefore honoring the cycle of life. Everything happens in its time, or as my Vavó used to say, "está na hora," in Portuguese. *It is the hour.* She would say this when the time had come for anything from taking bread out of the oven to major life transitions in our family—babies born or elders passing. Shiva manipulates the destruction and creation of life with a cosmic dance to shake the universe.

Om mane padme hum:

This mantra is more associated with Tibetan Buddhism than yoga, but you'll sometimes see it depicted in written form or hear it played in yoga studios. The chant is associated with the bodhisattva (awakened one) of compassion, Avalokiteshvara. The vibration of the six syllables evokes a powerful response in the person who repeats it, beyond the literal meaning of the words, which comprise countless translations and interpretations. You know *om*. Meanwhile, *mane* means jewel. *Padme* refers to the symbolic lotus flower. *Hum* means that. In essence, the mantra encourages the mind to dwell in the "jewel of the lotus flower."

Lam, vam, ram, yam, ham, sham, om:

These are all the sounds associated with each of the chakras that you learned in the previous section. Chant the sounds together, and feel the balancing and energy-boosting effect they have on your whole being. This is called the bija mantra. Some traditions use *om* for the third eye and silence as the sound associated with the crown chakra. I've included *sham* as the third eye sound and om for the crown, as taught to me by Deepak Chopra.

Lokah samastha sukhino bhavanthu:

The translation of this mantra is may all beings everywhere be happy, peaceful, and free. Because it has more of a direct translation than some of the others, it can be pronounced easily and enjoyed in English. It's a great one for children, who have fun considering all beings—people, animals, butterflies, polar bears—acting happy, peaceful, and free. My favorite memory of this mantra was when a teacher trainee of mine, Claire, had to lead me through a short yoga sequence for practice, as if I were her student. She'd had the bad luck of being paired with me rather than one of her peers and was very nervous. She did an excellent job, and when she concluded our mini session, she recited this mantra, only she misremembered it and instead said, "You are happy. You are peaceful. You are free." It made such an impression on me when expressed as a declaration rather than a wish. Claire went on to join the Peace Corps, working to improve health care in Rwanda for the next two years. It wasn't teaching yoga, and, yet, it was. She was a living, working embodiment of this mantra every day.

If Sanskrit feels intimidating or doesn't resonate with you like your mother tongue, you might try some English mantras. If another language rings truer and clearer for you than English, I encourage you to use it. Even after all those years in junior high, high school, and college French classes, I can only clumsily peck at words that flash cards left behind. My ears have a nostalgic familiarity with Portuguese from hearing it as a child, but my vocabulary is meager. Alas, English it is.

I am:

I used this mantra while teaching meditation to more than 300 executives at a business breakfast, and a year later, some of them still tell me how relaxed and focused it made them feel. They were in suits, possibly under- or overcaffeinated and anxious to start their workdays. Yet, they learned to savor the one time all day when they did not have to fill in the blank: I am a CEO. I am a parent. I am in a meeting. I am running late. Take time to just *be, with your infinite Self*, and *leave open* infinite possibilities.

I am _____ [fill in the blank].

When you need a certain form of energy or strength, it's helpful to state it clearly and repeatedly to wire its intention into your mind and body. It also helps to make statements in the present rather than future tense. Examples: I am strong. I am clear. I am light. I am peaceful. I am calm. I am love. I am enough.

Fortune favors the bold.

I wear this one, written in Latin (its original language) by Virgil, on a necklace. It's a great reminder when I need a small dose of courage.

Just. This.

Is it me, or do these two words perfectly capture the entire essence of mindfulness? The meditation center I bike to in Cambridge is open to the public in the mornings, and the sittings are unguided, meaning a teacher is there to unlock the center and sound the gong when our forty-five minutes is complete. Beyond that, there's no instruction. On occasion, the teacher shares a gem of Buddhist thought in the form of a mantra after the gong. *Just this* profoundly moved me when I first heard it. No matter where we are or what we are feeling, we can benefit from the subtle encouragement to focus on JUST. THIS. This moment, right here. Start with that. Live in that. It influences and improves all the other moments.

I also polled my OGs (om gals and guys who take my classes or follow me online) for their favorite mantras. Here is some of what they generously shared:

> Grace over perfection.
> Done is better than perfect.
> I am enough. I have enough. I do enough.
> I trust the timing of my life.
> Change happens now.
> Enlightenment is for everyone.
> Wings of angels.
> Dig deep.
> Be light.
> Be here now.
> I relinquish all regrets, grievances, and resentments.
> I thank god for making me the way I am.
> Thank you, _____.

Each mantra was declared with pride and shared with love, even the ones containing the f-bomb. (A striking number of people use mantras containing the f-bomb, I learned.) Which is OK, by the way. If it sparks something within you, if it fires you up, if it evokes your highest good (and obviously isn't meant or directed as an affront to anyone else's highest good), then you've found your mantra. *Eff yeah*, you have! A few friends shared these colorful examples:

- Harden the fuck up.
- Get all New York up in this b*tch.

Even as a Bostonian, I can respect this last one.

Tratak

If you've ever stared into a candle flame, watched a campfire crackle, or contemplated a small object like a photograph, flower, or statuette of a spiritual deity, you've unwittingly done *tratak* meditation. It's a useful way to hone attention, especially if closing one's eyes makes meditation more difficult as opposed to easier. For some people, closing their eyes makes them drowsy or mentally checked out. For victims of trauma, closing their eyes can flood them with unpleasant or scary memories and images. For these reasons and others, tratak can be a more user-friendly form of meditation.

Tratak means *to look* or *gaze upon* and describes a style of meditation in which yogis choose an object on which to meditate. Most often, this includes a candle flame. Other potential options could include a photograph of a loved one (perhaps someone who's passed on and you'd like to invite their spirit to sit with you); a memento from an inspirational place, such as a rock, seashell, or trinket; or a spiritual talisman. The goal is to let the mind settle through the help of the eyes. Ancient yogis established tratak as a sensory flushing for eyes. For modern yogis, it serves as a much-needed break from endless amounts of screen time each day. Just like our devices, we need to recharge. Of course there's no substitute for sleep, but tratak meditation is one easy way to recharge tired eyes and focus a mind that's low on energy any time of day. Just be sure to get your shut-eye at night.

Gratitude

The most direct route out of self-pity is gratitude, and the antidote to ego is counting one's blessings. Ego is born from a place of the small self, which feels scarcity, lack, and affronts to self-worth that lead us to say *What about me?* Gratitude is its enlightened and abundant counterpart—the big Self, which is deeply connected to all things and therefore unlimited in its capacity. As soon as you set the course for gratitude in your mind, it ripples through your whole being. When you are grateful for something outside yourself, you cannot remain small or scarce. The ego melts. The heart expands. The mind aligns with what is right rather than wrong with life, what is blessed and present, not missing or imagined.

Gratitude meditation is ideal for when you have those frustrating, prickly days of feeling sapped, swindled, or squashed by the world. Because we will all have these days. The key is catching ourselves before we go too far down the proverbial rabbit hole, using and developing the strength of our minds to gain better control of our inner environment, even in the most challenging times. The French painter Henri Matisse once declared, "Grace is an inner atmosphere." The following meditation is a beautiful example of creating grace within yourself whenever you need it.

As you breathe in, think to yourself, *Gratitude to* . . . As you breathe out, let images of people and experiences for which you are grateful come to you. Don't force it. Just witness what arises. By doing this meditation on a regular basis, you become better acquainted with your larger Self, the part of you that is connected to all things, as opposed to being at the mercy of the small self. Today, studies in social science and psychology verify what yogis have believed for centuries, which is that happiness is less dependent on external conditions and more commensurate with the levels of gratitude we contain and express within our lives.

Loving-kindness

The word *metta* represents the principle of loving-kindness, which is akin to the love a parent feels for a child. As you know from personal experience and countless romantic comedies, there are many forms of love. Metta is the unconditional kind that wants happiness for others independent of any self-interest. Buddhists seek to train this love like a muscle by exercising it. First, extend metta toward the self; next, offer loving-kindness to a beneficiary (someone who supports you); then, a loved one; neutral person (someone you neither like nor dislike); difficult person; and, last, an enemy. And you thought arm balances were hard!

Neuroscience offers evidence that our brains are impacted by meditation, citing evidence such as MRI scans that show heightened levels of activity in the brains of Buddhist monks, especially in the prefrontal lobes associated with compassion. The same areas of the brain are dim and underactive in the brains studied of hardened criminals. It's worth noting that the brain and the mind are two different things. For example, someone can have a genetic predisposition for addiction or high cholesterol but negate or vastly limit its impact by a different level of consciousness in the mind. The brain may want a drink or side of bacon, but the mind discerns otherwise. These enlightened choices rewire the brain, up or down—regulating patterns as deeply embedded in us as our genetic makeup. In other words, meditation practice can reshape our lives, from the inside out. Practice loving-kindness, through meditation and living, to fall in love with the gift of your life. You can sit quietly and absorb these heartfelt intentions for yourself and/or send them to anyone, anytime, anywhere in the world who needs them, and there is certainly no shortage of people and places in the world that need our loving-kindness right this minute. I recommend taking at least one, long, slow cycle of breath as you say each line aloud or to yourself.

May I be safe.
May I be happy.
May I be healthy.
May I live with ease.

May you be safe.
May you be happy.
May you be healthy.
May you live with ease.

No matter which style of meditation you choose, this practice does for your mind what asanas do for your body. With practice, the mind becomes stronger, more flexible, focused, and clear. Its decision-making center lights up. Its lower-functioning primal urges and outbursts abate. Through yoga, with its emphasis on mindfulness—the act of being present, on purpose, without judgment—the mind evolves into a kinder place to live. This benefit extends long past the end of a ninety-minute yoga class and beyond the edges of a mat.

Let's be candid, though: while its key principles are simple, meditation is not easy. By way of a confession, I fell off the meditation wagon around the holidays once. Funny visual, isn't it? I picture an actual wagon pulled by reindeer, through a snowy scene, with a bunch of people quietly meditating in the back. Then, I literally *fall off*. It makes one wonder, would people just shrug and continue meditating? I'd be left to gather myself, on a cobblestone street, dusting off the reindeer dung.

The actual story is less dramatic.

But it's a familiar one to many. We're on a roll with a healthy change—meditating, going to yoga or the gym, for example— until we miss a day. That day becomes a string of days, and soon, we've lost our mojo.

Mine came back at New Year's. (Also a familiar story—time of resolution and recommitment.) And I recommenced meditating each weekday morning thereafter. This time, it was the easiest and most enjoyable climb back on the wagon I've ever experienced. Not only did I regain momentum, my meditation practice didn't feel like a chore, which it can at times. Instead, I looked forward to it each morning and found it easy to carve out the time. Sounds crazy, right? What made it so easy? What had changed?

The answer is simple. The only thing that matters now is that I do it. I don't have to do forty-five minutes at my Buddha School in Cambridge at dawn. I don't have to do twenty minutes or even ten minutes. I just have to do it. Seven minutes? Wonderful. Five minutes is all I have? Fine. Forgive me for being a little thick, but this was a revelation at the time. Here I am writing a book about doing our om thing and I forgot to give myself enough leeway to do my own. So, I told my boyfriend, who you'll see obviously doesn't need yoga, when you hear how enlightened his response was.

"Isn't that the deal with anything? Do *something* . . . not nothing?"

There you have it, friends. If you're losing meditation mojo (or any healthy momentum for that matter) for any reason: do something; not nothing. Recalibrate your expectations a little. Do less, and see more of it, any of it, as progress in the right direction, from where you sit, back on the wagon.

....

A Meditation Practice of Your Om

....

- Each day, aim to meditate for ten minutes. Do this for ten days. Notice how you feel—not just during meditation but also throughout the day. How do you experience the highs and lows of a typical twenty-four hours? How do you sleep at night? Meditation itself doesn't feel all that different over time, but it has a drastic and cumulative effect on the rest of our lives as a whole.

- Each week, choose a daily task you do mindlessly—like unlocking a door, answering the phone, washing dishes, or logging in to your email. Turn it into a daily, real-world mindfulness practice. Do it consciously. Take a deep breath before getting started, and pay attention while doing it. Experience how the task and your perception of it change when you add awareness. Then, pick a new task.

- Each month, write down a new life-changing, love-filled intention in a centralized location—such as a calendar, plan book, to-do list, or journal. The act of putting your intention in writing prioritizes it. It may take more than a month to manifest, but that's OK. Remember, it's the feeling and focus your intention evokes within you that is most important. Some body, mind, and spirit suggestions:

  Embody _____ [fill in the blank].
  Work out hard. Work in easy.
  Stop waiting for someone to make you an expert at living your own life.
  Grace is my inner atmosphere.
  There is only love.

Om Expert:
Mallika Chopra, mother, meditator, founder of Intent.com, author of *Living with Intent*.

Her Om Thing:
The power of intention, as a way to anchor one's self in spirit and approach one's day with mindfulness, purpose, and joy.

What she says:
Intentions are our deepest desires that represent who we aspire to be and what values we want to embrace in our life. Intents

come from the soul, from that quiet place beyond thoughts and emotions. When we anchor our day with an intention, we set into motion the choices and situations to manifest it. For example, if my intent today is to appreciate the kindness of others, I will pay attention to the actions of others and feel more gratitude in my day. Or if I express the intent to meditate every day, then I may be more diligent about finding the time to do it. It is important to remember that we may waver from the path, but setting an intention helps guide us over time to live the life we want to live. I do recommend writing down your intents, in a journal or online, as the ritual of expressing it helps create momentum to realizing them.

How You Can Do It:

You can set an intention every morning, every week, throughout the day—whenever you are motivated to create that anchor for yourself. I love to set my intents after my meditation practice, but this is not necessary. Here is a short, simple meditation and intention-setting practice:

- Find a comfortable place to sit. There is no need to sit in a particular position, and if you need to adjust your position during the meditation, go ahead and do so.
- Close your eyes and take a few deep breaths to settle in to the moment.
- Mentally repeat "I AM," and continue to repeat these words in your head. There is no need to force concentration. You will notice that your mind begins to wander away from the words. This is normal. When you notice that your mind has wandered to other thoughts or noises in the environment, gently bring your attention back to the words "I AM."

- Ideally set aside fifteen minutes for this practice. However, if you can only do it for five or ten minutes, that too is fine.
- Come out of the meditation by no longer repeating the words "I AM." With your eyes still closed, take a few deep breaths.
- Now, set your intent for the day. Do not feel you have to think hard about the intent or that it has to be something important or monumental. Just listen to the thoughts that arise in your mind, and choose an intent that will give you joy, balance, and inspiration for the day.
- Open your eyes.
- If you are inspired, write your intention in a journal or post it on Intent.com. There is no need to share it, but some people do find that getting support from others gives momentum and meaning to their intent. Others like to keep it private to give their intents sanctity and their own space to blossom.

Part Four

The Spirit

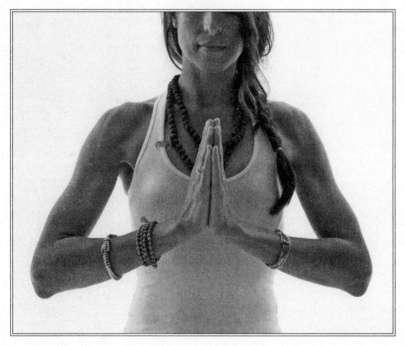

CHAPTER 9

OMG, Is Yoga Religious?

Spirituality has come a long way from the sanctity of churches and other traditional houses of worship. Today, it's broadly defined, practiced, and experienced in uniquely personal and modern ways, through everything from meditation apps to boutique spin classes. When it comes to yoga, an "exercise" class with deeply spiritual roots, there's a lot of confusion and controversy. All of which begs the question: does contemporary yoga honor its spiritual tradition? And should it? I believe it should, not just out of respect for the tradition of yoga but also for the genuine health and wholeness of our own lives and spirits.

We know that the tradition of yoga was born in India, even if most of us practicing yoga in the West were born far from there. Sometimes yoga's origins get the cultural respect they deserve. Sometimes they don't, especially if the business, entertainment, or sex appeal of yoga is given top priority. Often, yoga's ancestry is the root of some confusion for modern yogis. People tend to either idealize the cultural tradition (along with Hinduism) or reject its Eastern origins altogether. Either way, modern yogis are prone to feeling like they're doing it wrong—with some feeling as though they are never "Indian" enough, healthy enough, or spiritual enough, and others disregarding its heritage outright.

Of course, the best way to resolve these issues is to be open-minded and inquisitive about yoga's past, present, and future and to strive for authenticity of body, mind, and spirit in our inner and outer lives. Now that we've covered how yoga can help us heal the body and focus the mind, let's turn our attention to the realm of the soul—and how you can embrace the spiritual practice of yoga in your own way.

The Religion Question

We know that the foundation of yoga is spiritual, and the practice of it—with its eight limbs and many incarnations—aims to connect us to our spirits and/or to God. However, yoga is not a religion, and the tradition of yoga is not concerned with defining any one God. Instead, it offers us a path to feeling whole and alive, in whatever form that takes for each of us.

It's only when we're insecure about who we are, what we believe, or what we're practicing that we become anxious or judgmental about how others choose to live. This is true for all expressions of life, from yoga to parenting, worshipping God to going vegan. When the spirit is content, it doesn't need to meddle with or judge others. So, how can yoga make our spirits more content?

It's easier said than done, particularly when our regular yoga practice is more focused on fanciful physical forms than spirituality. Add busy, chronically booked-to-the-hilt schedules to the mix, and it's no wonder we feel disconnected. Who has time to make yoga more meaningful when I am lucky to get to class at all? The truth is that we don't need more time in our day to strengthen our spirits and let the inner journey unfold. We only need more awareness—time each day to consider and care for our spiritual health.

Some of us already have a well-defined spiritual practice, and we'd prefer to keep our yoga separate from our spirituality. There's nothing wrong with this approach. Yoga is plenty healthy this way. It's fun. It makes us more flexible and calm. It offers what you need when you need it. The only problem is that there's a strong possibility you might look up one day after calling yoga "just a workout" and realize you've been standing under the ceiling of the Sistine Chapel and calling it "just a ceiling." Yoga takes on new depth and artistry when it's grounded in soulful awareness. This can happen at any point, and you just might find yourself awestruck by the new view. Do yoga long enough, and I can promise you'll be awestruck many times.

Yogis might feel uneasy about the spiritual aspects of the practice for a variety of reasons. These include but are not limited to concern that practicing yoga conflicts with one's religion or faith, a preference to steer clear of the potential incense smoke and Hindu gods and goddesses present in some yoga studios, and, for people who do not believe in a higher power at all, the desire to avoid any reference to God (especially during their workout). These are all valid points, and we don't need to convert faiths, forgo fitness, or embrace a concept of God that does not suit us. As yogis, our main objective is to keep an open mind—like the gate of my meditation center—to elevate our awareness and feel a sense of oneness. Above all, yoga is meant to unify and connect, never divide or isolate. No matter how or where you start, the spirit cannot help but perk up with practice.

People connect to their divinity through yoga every day. Sometimes, we're in a pose on our mats or sitting in meditation and we're thinking about what's for dinner or the latest cliff-hanger episode of our favorite TV show. But, sometimes, we also think about big, existential questions like who we are and why we're here. We may experience glimpses of clarity about these things. It may occur to us that our heart is talking to us all day long. In yoga, we take a moment to listen intently. While I was writing this book, I confess that I got tired of yoga sometimes. I'd become overwhelmed, cranky, or even weepy on my kitchen floor. Any writer can attest that the amount of bad writing required to unearth good writing can be exhausting. Ditto all the research. I swore I didn't want to think or talk about yoga for one more nanosecond. Then—wouldn't you know it? I'd end up on my mat. I swear it wasn't by choice. It was like a yoga blackout. I'd come to in Half Pigeon and think *how the hell did I get here?* I'd breathe in deeply and out again. I'd notice the details of the experience of the moment—the coolness of the wood floor, the rise and fall of my breath, the hum of the dishwasher. I'd feel better. In the eighteen years I've been doing yoga, I've never once left my mat feeling worse. My spirit has never gotten heavier. I don't always achieve clarity or bliss—far from it—but that's still quite a record. I've never once rolled up my mat and been less convinced of the presence of some higher power.

To you, God may answer to Father, Allah, Christ, Goddess, or Hey-Up-There-If-You're-Listening. Its presence may feel like "love with a capital 'L,'" as Anne Lamott writes in her book *Help, Thanks, Wow: The Three Essential Prayers*, or the transcendent, Thoreauvian feeling you experience in nature. For many people, across many faiths, spending time in nature inspires a deeper level of consciousness or connection to spirit. In these moments, life makes sense (even the crummy parts), which is why people call them *aha* or *mountaintop* moments. When you're flanked by a forest or overlooking a shimmering body of water, it is hard not to think that things are connected in some divine way. However you experience these moments, they are opportunities for you to reunite with the version of *you* that matters most, the one independent of your hard-won or overlooked job title, killer or ho-hum outfit, swank or modest address, fabulous or utilitarian car, appearance, hair day, or changing thoughts or emotions. This core of who you are is peaceful, light, and true. It is your spirit and the part of you that bows to the same quality in all other beings at the end of yoga class. We've gotten really good at saying namaste. What's more essential and empowering is living it.

My Guru

My Vavó was my greatest spiritual teacher and a cornerstone of my faith, even as my spiritual path took very different turns from hers. I grew up Catholic like her but became a yogi (and a feminist to boot). I studied and strongly related to Buddhism. Hinduism fascinated me. Yet, whenever I grappled with my spiritual identity, as many of us do, I never needed to look too far beyond her example to find my answers. Was I a bad yogi if I ate her homemade kale soup—the first solid food she fed any of her grandchildren—because it contained meat? Did I forfeit the entire faith in which I was raised if I vehemently support gay and reproductive rights? Was I what my friend Joslyn calls a "half-assed Buddhist"? Most likely, yes, in terms of the last question, but I'm OK with that since Joslyn includes herself in this description, and Buddhists are so open-minded anyway. There's also a chance I was a better Buddhist in a past life and am still figuring it out in this one. Stand by; I'll let you know.

My point is that my grandmother's spirit was so strong and present that it showed me how life itself is a spiritual practice, that God can just as easily be found dancing in the kitchen on a Saturday morning (something my Vavó did frequently while baking bread and singing along to the Portuguese radio station), as in church on Sunday, as on a yoga mat any day of the week. I remember her skillfulness with seeing the sacred within the ordinary when I think of the following teaching by Gary Snyder:

> *All of us are apprenticed to the same teacher that the religious institutions originally worked with: reality. Reality insight says . . . master the twenty-four hours. Do it well, without self-pity. It is as hard to get the children herded into the carpool and down the road to the bus as it is to chant sutras in the Buddha-hall on a cold morning. One is not better than the other, each can be quite boring, and they both have the virtuous quality of repetition. Repetition and ritual and their good results come in many forms. Changing the filter, wiping noses, going to meetings, picking up around the house, washing dishes, checking the dipstick—don't let yourself think these are distracting you from your more serious pursuits. Such a round of chores is not a set of difficulties we hope to escape from so that we may do our "practice" which will put us on a "path"—it is our path.*

Finding what works for your spirit is an ongoing process and adventure. I wasn't always at peace with my path or able to access my own spirit. I had to think about what makes my life (and yoga) spiritual. I had to examine the faith into which I was born, including its shortcomings. I had to educate myself about other religions and foregoing religion altogether. I had to think about what honored my spirit, and what made it feel nourished and integrated into the rest of my life. I thought about all the ways one can talk to God. And all the ways you can walk through the world as a yogi.

Before she fell ill, when the flickers of dementia were few or only discerned after the fact, I had an *aha* moment with my grandmother. We were sitting outside on the deck of my parents' house, "getting sun on our legs" and chatting in our own language: part English, part Portuguese, all heart. Vavó wasn't much for sunbathing, but she liked to cuff her pants and feel the sun warm her shins. My nose was, as usual, buried in a book. Inside, something bubbled on the stove. Suddenly, Vavó wanted my attention.

"Habecca!" she said with urgency, pronouncing my name as she always did. My head jerked up from my reading.

"Yes, Vavó?"

"GOD . . ." she said, waving a finger in my direction and pausing for dramatic effect. This was going to be good, I knew. Funny, heartfelt, possibly crazy . . . maybe all three.

"God don't sleep," she declared.

It can be like this with Alzheimer's. Truth crystallizes into a more pure form, and the extraneous junk falls away. On the other hand, the shuffled information and lost memories can be like the stray keys you find floating in the bottom of a kitchen drawer. Where do they go? Who knows what they open anymore? For me, this insight clicked, like a spiritual skeleton key that opens many doors.

Whatever God is to you, whatever your spirit most revels in or feels inspired by, it doesn't sleep. It doesn't take a day off. It doesn't put a Do Not Disturb sign on the door, and if you email it, you won't get an Out of Office message. Thomas Merton once wrote, "Life is this simple: we are living in a world that is absolutely transparent, and God is shining through it all the time." This doesn't mean that life won't be difficult or painful, characterized by change and loss; it means that a higher power, the wellspring for your spiritual life, whether you realize it or not, is holding a candlelight vigil or perhaps a roaring bonfire for you all hours of the day and night. It doesn't sleep. It doesn't leave. It's always at the ready, and yoga is simply one more way of noticing and nourishing this fire, basking in its warmth, or letting it ignite and illuminate what you are most passionate about. Of the thing that most alights our spirits, my friend Vinita's mom likes to say that *God is the thing that moves people.*

God is goodness. It's love with a capital L and the feeling you get when you look at a sky full of stars, mountain chains, or giant waves. It's being a living Buddha or Christ or meeting one in a hospital waiting area, working late at an inner-city school, serving meals in a homeless shelter, or keeping warm at a bus stop in winter. It's Shiva, the destroyer, or St. Rita of impossible feats. That was my grandmother's name, Rita.

Stretching Your Spirit

Before we dive in further, let's be clear about something: I'm not a religious scholar or proselytizer. The last thing I want to do is tell someone else about his or her spirit. My hope, then, is to share ways of connecting to it and personalizing your yoga path, rather than to share a vision of the Promised Land as I see it, from my own experience. In drawing from my course of study and professional work with thousands of students over many years, I only offer observations and suggestions for finding spiritual sustenance in your life, when you need it, with a little help from yoga.

Ralph Waldo Emerson believed that everyone should make his/her own bible. "Select and collect all the words and sentences that in all your readings have been to you like the blast of a trumpet," he advised. Likewise, I believe you should collect and curate your yoga. This is what it means to do your om thing. I hearken back to yoga tradition not because I am an expert on the subject like the late Georg Feuerstein or scholar Mark Singleton or because I think it's the "better" yoga but because I value its inspiration. There's a lot of wisdom awaiting us in teachings stemming from centuries ago, and their relevance is underrepresented in ways that feel accessible or, dare I say, *fun* to modern yogis. We've gotten very good at making yoga more exercise driven and entertaining, with various accoutrements, music, and fashion trends. However, these additions often come at the sacrifice of something else, namely yoga's spiritual component. Therefore, this section poses questions of self-reflection and offers suggestions for spiritual sustenance through yoga *without* needing accoutrements or even a mat.

I love yoga philosophy, and studying it has enriched my practice over the past eighteen years. I'd even go so far as to say it's the glue that holds together my inner and outer lives. I also enjoy how yoga tradition overlaps with two faiths that originated in the same geographic location of India. When they are woven together as inspirations or in practice, a rich tapestry emerges. Yet, Hinduism and Buddhism are not one and the same, nor should they be confused with yoga. None of them are interchangeable, just as Bikram yoga is hot, but not all hot yoga is Bikram. Some yogis throughout the world are Hindu or Buddhist, but doing yoga does not make one Hindu or Buddhist. Historically, these spiritual paths cross-pollinated each other, frequently sharing sacred texts, symbols, vocabularies, and values. Today, if nothing else, they share some workshop programming at your average yoga retreat center. And although it's extremely difficult (even for qualified scholars) to date spiritual traditions that originated and evolved orally—many millennia before the written word or the birth of Christ—the consensus is that Hinduism began between 3000 and 1300 BCE, and while yoga, as we know it today, is quite new, its origins date back as far as the Vedas, the oldest Hindu texts (1500 to 1000 BCE). Meanwhile, the Buddha lived around 400 BCE. Yoga changed imperceptibly during some periods and rapidly in others, as it is doing now.

The final frontier of the yoga journey is its *spiritual stretching*. Yoga spreads out and starts touching more corners of your life, like a studio apartment in which one can simultaneously lie in bed, turn on the shower, and cook an omelet. I've plucked some of my favorite inspirations from yoga tradition, which I offer as suggestions for spiritual sustenance. Choose only what works for you, and feel free to add your own "spiritual stretches." If there's one trademark of modern yoga, it's the creativity of people who experimented and evolved an existing practice into something new. According to Mark Singleton, author of *The Yoga Body*, modern yoga, as we know it, arose when Indians began experimenting and merging forms of European gymnastics and wrestling with traditional yoga practices such as pranayama, dharana, and meditation. This theory seemed like heresy to some people, but the rich, complex history of yoga only further suggests that it is meant to offer the path we need when we need it. It also seems to caution yogis (albeit gently and maybe over a cup of tea) that our actions should reflect our priorities when it comes to the next stage of evolution for modern yoga. Should it be comprised largely of expensive products and yoga celebrity or, perhaps, something else? If the spiritual element of yoga speaks to you, it's helpful to understand why. If you like the feeling when yoga follows you off the mat, then it's time to learn how to create that state within yourself more often.

To this end, I'll frame the suggestions for spiritual sustenance around some of the deities who regularly appear in yoga iconography, not because you need to start worshipping them, convert to Hinduism, or because you need to know who they are to be a "real yogi," but because what they symbolize captures a slice of all our lives. They represent universal truths to which anyone of any faith can relate. They're archetypes that might infuse your yoga and life with a glint of inspiration or a *breath of spirit* if you will. We'll focus on the deities who appear most often, including but not limited to those whose images are frequently seen in yoga studios, the icons featured in clothing and jewelry designs, and as namesakes of poses we regularly practice, like Hanumanasana (splits) or Natarajasana (Dancer's Pose), for example. Of course we are always free to see postures strictly as physical maneuvers of flexibility and fitness and nothing more. Or, they are starting points to something bigger, deeper, and more sacred for which you're now ready. It's for you to decide.

CHAPTER 10

Suggestions for Spiritual Sustenance

I chose nine suggestions for spiritual sustenance because nine is a
factor of 108, which is a sacred number in yoga. There are said to be
108 *marmas* or sacred points on the body, 108 *pithas* or sacred places
in India, and 108 primary Upanishads, a sacred text and one of the
earliest places in writing in which yoga is revealed. (*The Bhagavad
Gita* is the most well-known of its stories.) The number has significance in astronomy, too, with 108 corresponding to the average distance of the Sun, Earth, and Moon being 108 times their respective
diameters. And mala beads, mentioned earlier as a tool for mantra
meditation like a rosary or worn as stylish accessories (being spiritual and stylish need not be mutually exclusive), traditionally contain 108 beads. This is how you can tell if the beads you bought were
intended for meditation or fashion. All sacred symbolism aside, one
of my favorite associations with the number 108 came in the form of
a very modern yogi moment, occurring—where else?—online, when
a former student, now talented teacher in Philadelphia, tweeted:

"108 emails in my inbox. I think it's a sacred sign . . . that I procrastinate email reading."

Each spiritual tradition has its own sacred numbers. The number ten, referring to the Ten Commandments, plays an important role in the sacred traditions and rituals of Christianity, Judaism, and Islam. Seven is also significant to these religions: there are the mythic seven days of creation in Christianity, seven days of sitting shivah to honor the passing of a loved one in the Jewish faith, and seven levels of Heaven for Muslims. In Hinduism, there are seven sages, known as the *saptarishi*, some of whom have yoga poses named for them, such as Visvamitrasana and Vasisthasana. Buddhism has its four Noble Truths and eight-fold path. Numbers often help us put some order to the contents of a spiritual life. Though they are finite, they help us express the infinite.

Repetition and ritual help ground our days and demarcate trails for our souls to travel, which is why they're hallmarks of all spiritual traditions. When the mind is quiet, consumed in a ritualized task, the soul can take over. By focusing the mind on repeating or enumerating something, the spirit becomes more available and capable of contemplation and wonder. No matter how busy we are, we can count the ways our spirit is alive. We can focus energy on something small but meaningful within our day, and in doing so, deepen our connection to self and Spirit.

An easy way to begin your meditation practice is to incorporate a favorite or lucky number. Try repeating a mantra a certain number of times or meditate for a set number of minutes. When plans fell through to go on a meditation retreat for New Year's Eve, my friend and I created our own retreat by attending a yoga class, enjoying a healthy dinner, then meditating for twelve minutes and doing a journaling exercise where we wrote down twelve things we wanted to release at midnight of 2012. Befitting the exercise, we burned the list (in a fire-safe bowl). I also love marking birthdays with special numbers. I do yoga on my birthday, incorporating my new age into the number of sun salutations or meditation minutes. Patricia Walden regularly does the number of dropbacks (from a standing position to wheel pose) that correspond to her age. She's now more than sixty-five years old. When her guru, B.K.S. Iyengar, turned eighty-five, she did eighty-five. Yes, I'm serious. That's the only way to talk about Iyengar folks; they are dead serious about their yoga (lovably so). Naturally, smaller numbers are more efficient; larger numbers require more time or skill with whatever you're doing.

The suggestions that follow incorporate lessons from traditional yoga philosophy, including the rich symbolism behind the gods and goddesses most frequently found in yoga today. Again, this is not the same as worshipping these deities or practicing Hinduism. Instead, they're mythic inspirations handed down to teach us about yoga and ourselves: anytime, anywhere. Many people consider the dieties to be representations of aspects of ourselves. Hindus believe that there is one God-energy, which takes many forms, represented by the deities. Similarly, there's one yoga with countless ways of practicing. I hope these suggestions inspire yours.

9 Suggestions for Spiritual Sustenance

1. Create. Sustain. Let Go.

You are a yogi in the information age, faced with incessant connectivity, automated everything, and seductive social media options every moment of the day. Most of us juggle schedules that yogis mere decades ago would find dizzying. Today, it's unlikely you have an Indian guru or ashram. You have a boss who wants that proposal on her desk by 5:00 p.m. and a sinking suspicion that the translation of ashram is something along the lines of *place for caffeine-withdrawal headache made worse by chanting.*

Yet, instead of prioritizing meditation or spiritual connection to soothe our stress at the end of a long day, it's still easier to drink red wine, eat dark chocolate, and lose ourselves in an addictive TV show about someone else's more enthralling, doomed, or glamorous life while scrolling Facebook looking at photos of someone else's seemingly more enthralling, doomed, or glamorous life. It's easier to *lose ourselves*. Period.

It's easier, more immediately gratifying, and better sold as society's hype. But don't buy the hype! It never works. If, for example, I regularly choose to smooth the edges off a tough day with a couple glasses of Malbec, the brainless comfort of TV, and safe distance of interacting with people largely online, without much interest or investment in practicing genuine coping skills for what makes a day—or string of days—tough, I know that my spirit suffers. I'm relying on outward sources to do an inside job. And these small avoidances of my inner environment on a difficult day are amplified over time and fall even shorter when the really challenging and traumatic life stuff hits, which it does for all of us at some point.

There's a popular Zen saying that the easy path leads to the hard life, and the hard path leads to the easy life. Modern life's easiest path is one that supports and valorizes high-speed distraction, disconnection, entertainment, avoidance, numbing, or shielding by any means necessary. If we're not careful, we can stay distracted every hour of every day, while our wholeness remains unknown to us. Modern yoga, by extension, can reinforce or release the energy behind these choices. It's possible to use yoga to both contort and compete or choose a more awakened and compassionate way of life.

The way of greater ease and spiritual connection requires choosing a different path, which may be harder in the short term. Over time, however, it's more conducive to the stronger spirit, which handles adversity with grace and connects deeply to the world around it. This isn't woo-woo; this is a fundamental truth of life. We get good at what we practice, and most of us are getting very good at half paying attention to our lives. Even in yoga classes, more and more people are practicing keeping one eye trained to their cell phones, discreetly placed just aside their mats, perhaps camouflaged by a towel. If we repeatedly dodge who we are and what we feel by accessorizing each spare moment with outside stimulus, we only get more adept at looking outside ourselves. If we practice living our lives for others—our parents, partners, or society—it becomes harder to remember what it feels like to authentically be ourselves. Yoga reminds us.

Brahma, Visnu, and Shiva are the three most prominent gods in Hinduism, so they have some influence over yoga tradition. For example, as much as yoga has evolved and as many styles that exist, we all end classes in Savasana, also known as Shiva's pose, he being the Lord of Destruction. When you rest in Savasana at the end of class, you're not taking a nap or lazing aimlessly on the floor. You're honoring the deepest core of your being and letting go of everything else. Here's a bit more on these powerful deities, along with the spiritual lessons they teach about creating, sustaining, and letting go, the beginning, middle, and end of all our endeavors on and off the mat.

Create.

Brahma is known as the supreme creator. When you begin a healthy habit; try a new style of yoga; show up for your first day on the job or at school, gleaming with possibility, attention sharpened like fresh pencils; or have the early conversations of a new romance or friendship with the same honesty and compassion you hope characterize it later, you nod to Brahma. You practice the "art of the start." You create anew. Create a life. Create a family. Create a business plan. Concoct a new recipe, or write the first page of the first chapter. The energy of Brahma is with you and within you. It's how you prepare and invoke each new stage of your journey.

As many of us can attest, getting started is often the hardest part, like getting out of bed and showing up to a 6:00 a.m. yoga class; asking someone on a first date; or admitting you need help to battle depression, addiction, or an eating disorder. It takes courage to begin, but it gets easier. Yogis seek to prepare the best conditions for success, and then it's a matter of repetition, momentum, and perseverance. At the core of a meaningful life is the desire and capacity to take the steps needed to create what we want.

Om Work: Visualize

Visualize a new opportunity or life goal that you want to create. Perhaps it's a healthy habit, loving relationship, career milestone, artistic creation, or daring yoga pose. Invite the energy of Brahma to help you. See what this new beginning looks like. Where are you when it happens? What are you wearing? How does the moment feel? What mindset, muscles, resources, or people do you need to start? Set the scene in your mind so realistically that your body believes you've been there.

Om Expert:
Kim Vandenberg, U.S. Olympic medalist in swimming.

Her Om Thing:
Creative visualization, a technique that anyone can use to harness the power of the mind.

What she says:
Visualization techniques have been proven time after time to breed success. Someone once told me there is a difference between racing to win and racing not to lose. I was lucky to have a coach during my teenage years who introduced our team to visualization. He would guide us in this form of meditation in the weeks leading up to our big races. We would gather by the walls, put our legs up while lying on our towels, and close

our eyes. Step by step, we would imagine every detail of the environment, the more specific the better. We would imagine the natatorium, our warmups, what suit we were wearing, what the water temperature was, how many people were in our lanes. Stroke by stroke, we would see ourselves and feel ourselves swimming, breathing, kicking, and finishing our races strong. We would pay attention to every detail. Often, our heart rates would increase and our breathing would quicken; our bodies were reacting to our thoughts. The power of the mind is a tool used in practically every sport; however, it can easily be transferred to daily nonathletic life by bringing comfort and confidence to situations in which we feel stress and pressure. Seeing is believing.

How to do it:

- Choose a comfortable and restorative yoga pose, such as Savasana or Viparita Karani (Legs-up-the-Wall Pose).
- Close your eyes and breathe deeply.
- Listen inward, to the space between your breaths, to your heartbeat, to your intuition.
- Then, begin to mentally walk yourself through an important life event. It doesn't have to be Olympic caliber—just something that inspires you to be your best self.
- Visualize every detail of the environment; what it looks like, what you're wearing, who is nearby, how you feel, which sounds, scents, and sights characterize this moment, and how you move your body.
- Finally, see your highest good and greatest level of achievement in this moment. Remember, anything anyone has ever accomplished began, first, as a thought.

Sustain.

According to the *Yoga Sutras*, two qualities are needed for wholeness: *abhyasa* (practice/discipline) and *vairagya* (letting go). Along
with Brahma's help at the start, Visnu, known as the sustainer of the
universe, inspires us to cultivate the discipline needed to continue,
preserve, succeed, and see our commitments through. When we fall,
we'll rise with his help or the energy he symbolizes.

Known to Hindus as the god of preservation, Visnu is the sustaining force that carries the torch for Brahma. Because the fresh
idea or bold beginning needs backup and nurturing to fully develop.
After we take the initial step, score the date, or arrive on our first
day at the office with shiny shoes and big ideas, then what? Can we
deliver? Do we have staying power, persistence, patience, and resilience when things don't go as planned (because they rarely do)? How
will we stoke our creativity, execute our ideas, and nurture our relationships? Most of all, how will we react to inevitable missteps and
faltering?

There's a Zen proverb, which I love, that speaks to this spiritual
lesson of tenacity: "Six times down, seven times up." Before you quit
or concede, maybe make this your new mantra. Certainly, there are
times when we need to know when to let go (and we'll talk about that
next), but when it comes to creating and sustaining what we value
most, Brahma and Visnu embody that inspiration and fortitude. Remember, to understand or invite these energies into your yoga practice is not the same as religious worship, it's simply an opportunity
to tap into archetypes we all experience, universal truths that guide
us on our spiritual paths.

When you think about Visnu energy in your life, consider what
sustains you. What do you want to make room for, and who helps you
do this? The following exercise can help you stay the course or free
up renewed energy to keep going when you falter.

Om Work: Write

Write down a list of people, places, and things that sustain you. Keep this list close when you feel like quitting.

Conversely, what's one thing you need to *stop* doing right now so that you free up energy for something more essential? It can be a hard lesson to learn, especially if you're a people pleaser like me, but saying NO is often an important way of saying YES to something better.

Let Go.

Vinyasa yoga classes (the most popular style of yoga offered in the United States at the time of publication and what I predominantly teach) flow with a signature cadence, an iambic pentameter of yoga sequencing. Some teacher-training programs encourage aspiring teachers to consider the three-pronged godhead of Brahma, Visnu, and Shiva as an efficient way to prepare, guide, and conclude their classes, like the one I led in Boston with its curriculum created by Allison English and Alanna Kaivalya for Pure Yoga.

For instance, Brahma represents the preparation of the class, including planning the sequence (which poses or parts of the body will be emphasized), adjusting the room temperature, perhaps lighting incense and playing music as students arrive, and generally making them feel welcome by setting a tone and mood in the studio. The teacher might encourage students to set an intention for their practice (although this is something students can always do regardless of whether a teacher prompts it). Then, momentum builds, as if inspired by Visnu's powers of preservation. A good teacher is holding the students' attention, and since their bodies are warmer now that they've been moving, it's the ideal stage to pepper in more challenging poses. If the teacher threads a philosophical theme through the class, it is maintained here, the theme and sequence illuminating one another. This is a key way to underscore that a pose's appearance isn't the priority but rather its attitude. When you're in a yoga class like this one, created and sustained so deliberately, you know something special is happening. The teacher is like a sherpa, guiding you up a mountain. Finally, the class winds down. Poses are more cooling and restful toward the end, eventually closing with Savasana, Shiva's pose, also known as Corpse Pose. With any luck, this miniature ritual destroys the psychic debris of the day. We shed the roles we played. We quiet the frenetic mind. We soften some anxiety; we heal the spiritual fatigue. What remains is our innermost self, stripped clean and laid bare, like fresh-tilled earth. This is the pivotal lesson of Shiva: from the end of something—a long day, yoga class, relationship, or job—something new can grow stronger and healthier than previously possible.

Om Work: Reflect

Think about a time when you ended something efficiently or even positively. You outgrew a habit, graduated from school, left a relationship, moved on from a job, or said good-bye to a loved one passing on without leaving anything unsaid or unfinished. Honoring endings and deaths is a way to respect the cycle of life, just as Savasana honors the end of a yoga class. Above all, don't forget to let your yoga and life journey assimilate, land, and recharge you through the power of Savasana. It's such a simple, powerful, and fertile time for your body, mind, and spirit to connect and rest deeply. Don't miss it.

We are what we repeatedly do, said Aristotle. Like Brahma, Visnu, and Shiva, we learn to honor the beginning, middle, and end of all things through yoga. We create, sustain, and let go. And the more we practice, the better we get at accepting and evolving through these stages, the less time we spend distracted or lost from ourselves. Which is to say the better we get at trusting and fully participating in the process of life.

2. Be You Bravely.

To deepen my yoga practice, I read the *Bhagavad Gita*. I was in college when I realized it was an important text in yoga tradition, one of the first places in print in which we hear about yoga. So, I bought a copy, read it, highlighted the lines I liked best, and dog-eared the heck out of its pages. More than a decade later, I keep it atop my stack of most referenced yoga books. It still acquires new highlights and dog-ears.

The first time I read the *Gita*, I was surprised by its subject matter. There I was, a developing yogi and coed to boot, and therefore doubly wide-eyed and idealistic, expecting an inspiring message about peace and love. I had no idea that the *Gita* is an epic tale of war, 700 verses that are part of a larger ancient text called the *Mahabharata*. I felt confused. What ruse was this? It was like signing up for gentle tai chi and getting mixed martial arts fighting instead. What happened to *ahimsa*? Where was the peace and love? How could the first mentions of yoga in print be in the context of a battle?

Simple, it turns out. Yogis (ancient and modern) relate to the allegory of battle. It's a familiar storyline, an archetype for life. The *Gita* is not about weapons and war tactics but our own interior warfare through the tale of its protagonist, the soldier Arjuna, and the counsel he receives from the god Krishna (an incarnation of Visnu). Like any story as timeless and heavily translated as the *Gita*, different themes prevail depending on the edition: which translation, in which language, and by whom. For some, it's a story of *dharma*: work or sacred duty. For others, it's about devotion, discipline, or selflessness. It's all of these, of course. Naturally, it's also about bravery. I'm continually startled by how human and familiar Arjuna sounds as he shakes and quakes with fear, standing on the precipice of war. He tells Krishna:

My limbs sink,
My mouth is parched,

My body trembles,
The hair bristles on my flesh.

The magic bow slips
From my hand, my skin burns,
I cannot stand still,
My mind reels.

My translation? He's scared shitless. We all know this feeling, when our stomach drops and breath shallows. It's the stuff of public speaking, possible shark attacks, or the phone ringing in the middle of the night. No one escapes life without a generous share of their own real and imagined battles, and each time we face and triumph over fear in any small or epic expression, our spirit brightens. We become brave by seeing our battles clearly and courageously taking action. This is why Krishna persists. He pushes Arjuna. To be brave requires faith. It sustains us to nourish what we love rather than kowtow to what we fear. Not to mention that to be alive is to wage battle—even for yogis, as nonviolent or "granola" as we might appear. It's the essence of one of my favorite quotes by e.e. cummings:

> *To be nobody but yourself in a world which is doing its best, night and day, to make you everybody else means to fight the hardest battle which any human being can fight; and never stop fighting.*

In Brené Brown's best-selling book *Daring Greatly* and her top-ranked TED Talk, she shares the theory that our greatest potential, as people, parents, and leaders, is in our ability to face the fears that make us feel vulnerable, along with years of empirical data as a researcher in social work to back it up. If e.e. cummings creates poetry emblematic of our interior battle, Brené brings the real-life data. With a candid and compassionate voice, she outlines the importance of developing resilience to shame for the purpose of becoming whole. To describe people who believe they are deserving of love and connection (our most primal need) and are, therefore, better able to cope with the daily battle of being "nobody but yourself," she coins the term: the *Wholehearted*. This terminology, now shared with Oprah and on NPR, among other media outlets, bears an uncanny resemblance to the definition of yoga: to make whole.

"For a man without self-mastery, the self is like an enemy at war," cautions Krishna in the *Gita*. Inherently, we know we are our own worst critics and most daunting enemies. We see the weak, scared, or shameful parts of ourselves, and we don't want to face them. They make us quiver, like Arjuna. The spiritual lesson of daring greatly, doing yoga, and nourishing a strong spirit is to face our fears and take bold action. I borrowed the title of this lesson from my vivacious friend Jessica, who shared her personal mantra of spiritual sustenance with me in an email. *Be you bravely.* I looked at the words for a while, three of them standing there, and they cut to my core. "So sever the ignorant doubt in your heart with the sword of self-knowledge," says Krishna. Know yourself, even when it's scary, even when you must look into the dark corners of who you are, and be you bravely.

Finally, implicit in the lesson of being ourselves bravely is that we are not trying to be anyone else. Inspiration is all around, and feeling inspired or motivated by someone else is a magical and essential part of life and the creative process. Make no mistake: life is a creative process. But there's a difference between doing your om thing and ripping off someone else's. "You were born an original, don't die a copy," cautioned the artist John Mason. In other words, to be the hero of your own epic tale: be you bravely—and only you.

Om Work: Cultivate Bravery

Counsel Yourself with a Mantra:

Incorporate the mantra *be you bravely* into a japa meditation (see page 165), or make up your own bravery-bolstering phrase. Repeat it to yourself whenever the next small or epic battle arises. Set a reminder on your phone with these powerful words at a time when you suspect you will need them, such as before a scary doctor's visit, hard personal conversation, or important work meeting.

Do Something Scary:

Choose a yoga pose that scares you, such as an inversion, and practice it every day for at least seven days (or choose your own spiritual number of significance!). Notice what happens. Think about how this focus, tenacity, and courage could be directed to larger endeavors.

Apply Ancient Inspiration:

Write down a favorite quote from the *Bhagavad Gita* and post it somewhere prominent in your home. Look at it often and invite the timeless wisdom of those words to enter your day. Here are some of my favorites:

- *It is better to live your own destiny imperfectly than to live an imitation of somebody else's life with perfection.*
- *Look to your own duty. Do not tremble before it; nothing is better for a warrior than a battle of sacred duty.*
- *The power of God is with you at all times; through the activities of mind, senses, breathing, and emotions; and is constantly doing all the work using you as a mere instrument.*
- *No effort in this world is lost or wasted.*
- *Be forever lucid, alive to yourself.*
- *Be impartial to failure and success—this equanimity is called discipline.*
- *Without discipline, he has no understanding or inner power; without inner power, he has no peace; and without peace, where is joy?*

- *He should elevate himself by the self, not degrade himself; for the self is its own friend or its worst foe.*

Forgive Someone:

Forgiveness is brave. Not to mention healthy. Carrying around old grudges and grievances is like being exposed to any other form of toxin, like GMOs, BPAs, or too much TMZ. We can survive limited exposure, but too much and too frequently has negative long-term effects on our physical, mental, and spiritual health. There's a Buddhist teaching that when you hold on to anger, it is as if you are holding a hot coal with the intention of throwing it at someone. You are the one who gets burned. You don't need to invite the person to dinner, stay in the unhealthy relationship, or act Stepford sweet and phony. You do need to drop the grudge that's weighing you down and making you small. Be brave and move forward.

3. Believe in Abundance.

I know I was tough on the word *abundance* earlier. So, this is where I call a truce. It's not that I find the concept problematic. Not at all. Abundance is divine. Who doesn't love abundance?

What I don't love is the overuse and emptiness the word has acquired in today's yoga circles. It feels saccharin or hippy dippy when tossed around too much, especially if you've been doing yoga long past the honeymoon phase, even more so if you teach yoga.

The dirty little secret of working in the yoga industry is that it's a relentless hustle. Anyone who tells you otherwise is putting on airs or has an alternate source of financial income/support. After rising to the highest levels of the busiest yoga studio in the world, at that time, I found myself working so hard to make ends meet that I lived through two Boston winters without heat and lost my voice on a weekly basis due to overuse. To be fair, my roommate and I had space heaters. We turned on the oven often and baked brownies. We had the option of turning on the heat at any time, but we opted not to. We treated it as a friendly competition with Mother Nature. How long could we last? How tough could we be? But, let's be honest, it was a decision based on finances, not foolhardy fun. Most twentysome-things know some degree of these sacrifices well. Ditto victims of the "great recession," single parents, starving artists, bootstrapping entrepreneurs, and everyone else not part of a very small segment of the population who doesn't spend some time or a lifetime scrimping. And the voice. This was not a raspy, sexy, Scarlett Johansson situa-tion. This was opening my mouth and no sound coming out. People have reoccurring nightmares about this kind of thing. For me, it was a harsh reality.

I took my predicament to my manager, who suggested that I reflect upon my own role in what was becoming a chronic ailment and sug-gested I consider going to a "group therapy program" in Europe. To be clear, this wasn't vocal therapy. It was a pseudospiritual commu-nity with roots in 1970s est training seminars and flagged as a cult in much of the Internet research I did. To be doubly clear, flights to Europe are not cheap. It was an investment in my own abundance, I was told. I declined and instead went to a specialist at Massachu-setts General Hospital. When the elevator opened at the top floor of a glass building, a jovial man greeted me as if at a party rather than a doctor's appointment. I looked at his nametag. *Sunny*, it said. Makes sense, I thought. The diagnosis was fairly simple. I was using my voice so much, teaching nonstop and projecting it over a loud heating system used to heat the studio to over ninety degrees with ninety or so heavy-breathing humans in attendance each class, multiple times a day, every day of the week, that I'd developed lesions on my vocal cords. I could have surgery. But I was pretty sure my meager health insurance was not going to cover it, nor could I afford to take that much time off. So, here I was: doing a job I loved, at which I was good, yet feeling swallowed whole.

It was also around this time that I was dumped on the night of a funeral. When stated that way, it sounds morbid and overdramatic, but it happened. It took a long time to recover for both of us. A young man who loses a strong, graceful, single mother after a protracted illness can't be expected to fathom how to be in the world without her, not initially, at least. My ex knew he was headed into a dark place, and he refused to take me with him. (Of course I would end up in my own dark place.) I cried so hard I threw up. I prayed endlessly that he would come back. I went to church on my own volition for the first time. When fellow parishioners expressed concern over the fact that I seemed to be sniffling (OK, near sobbing) in the back row, I told them it was an allergic reaction to frankincense and scurried awkwardly to my car.

All this is to say that life in my midtwenties was not characterized by abundance, financially or spiritually. It was the least abundant, most scarce time in my life. I was broke and brokenhearted, and I needed to make changes. Eventually, I put back together my heart and finances. I regained my voice, in more ways than one. I realized that a life filled with "yoga" but devoid of balance wasn't sustainable for me anymore. I left the yoga industry for a period. In many ways, I left an old self and stepped into a new one. Life started to feel more abundant. The source of this abundance wasn't just the new job or steadier paycheck, of course. It was me. I could see myself as someone who did, indeed, have a role in my scarcity *and* my abundance. I didn't need a trip to Europe to tell me this. I made some smart investments of my most valuable currency, and things started to change, germinate, evolve, and expand.

Yoga and money have a precarious relationship. Like many spiritual practices, early depictions of yoga made being a yogi and attaining wealth mutually exclusive. Yogi ascetics, for example, shunned material possessions, wandered forests foraging for food, or relied on the generosity of nearby villagers to support them. For the modern yogi, that's less feasible and desirable. So, the jig is up about yoga and money. On its own, money is neither bad nor unspiritual.

It's simply another form of energy. You're on a spiritual path whether you know it or not. You need to pay your bills whether you want to or not. When the spiritual and material aspects of our lives feel abundant, we're better at managing them. When we operate from a place of scarcity, we feel just that: scarce. Our spiritual and material lives are equally capable of feeling indebted and lacking, and beyond that, feeling bereft in one area can easily overshadow the other.

The archetype tasked with areas of wealth and abundance, both material *and* spiritual, is the goddess Lakshmi. She reminds us of the universe's abundance and generous nature. She's the wife of Visnu, preserver of the universe, which is fitting since wealth is needed to maintain life, beginning with our most basic needs of food, water, and shelter (ideally heated in the winter). She's beautiful, adorned in a brightly colored sari trimmed in gold, as she travels by lotus flower (basically a throwback Prius). The image of the lotus flower, a beautiful blossom that grows out of the muddiest, murkiest waters is a prevalent one in yoga, as it symbolizes growth out of adversity. The flower doesn't grow *despite* the muck. It grows *because of* it, just as spiritual transformations so often come from our darkest, muddiest moments. Gold coins pour from Lakshmi's hands.

The coins are symbolic, of course, since money is only one form of currency, and it's not even our most valuable currency. As I learned firsthand and have mentioned before, our most valuable currency is our attention: how we think about ourselves and the world, our capacity for wealth of all kinds, and our investments of body, mind, and spirit. The most valuable real estate we own is not property but perspective, held within the space in our own minds. Think about it. Even the most posh beachfront property can wash away with a hurricane. A home can burn to the ground from a teetering candle. Meanwhile, nothing can reduce the value of your attention but you, and what you can create with the focus of your mind is immeasurable. The thing that sustains and prospers within you when all the external trappings fall away is true wealth. In turn, this energy can be channeled to create other forms of wealth, including but not limited to money. Invest attention lazily, begrudgingly, or aimlessly, and you'll find success, any way you choose to define it, harder to come by. Invest attention and intention consciously and it pays dividends.

No matter how modest or lavish your situation, do not be scared of thinking about your wealth. Consider, first, the areas in which you are abundant. For me, it was an education, set of skills and passions, and a group of friends who never let me buy into the fear that I didn't deserve better and couldn't change my situation. Then, expand upon what you have. How can you grow it? Who will help you? Last, see yourself through a Lakshmi lens. Put a picture of her somewhere in your home. See her beauty and brilliance. If her image doesn't work for you, choose someone or something else that reminds you of the universe's abundance. This isn't about how to be a perfect yogi or billionaire. It's about being the healthiest version of yourself that you can be, in all the ways one exudes physical and financial health. Here are some important questions to think about to guide you back to Lakshmi's energy when your material or spiritual balance feels low.

Om Work: Reflect

What does abundance mean to you?

What are the first things that come to mind? If you don't know what you're trying to create, how can you create it? What would abundance look and feel like *for you*?

What do you feel you're lacking in terms of abundance?

Financial wealth, rich friendships, strong family connections, rewarding work, enough sleep, enough education, enough intimacy with your partner, a loving partner? Think about the things that feel scarce and consciously take one small but immediate step toward depositing into your own emotional or fiscal bank account today.

What can you give up?

Overwhelmingly, research shows that once basic needs are met (i.e., food, shelter, safety), happiness no longer correlates with increases in financial wealth, largely because our standards continue to rise as well. The more we have, the more we want. In this way, regularly checking our desires is a healthful opportunity to maintain financial health. You don't have to give up your fine tastes, but discretion is important. It also adds value to the experience of fine things and splurges. This curbing of desires also applies to sneaky habits or behaviors that make us feel scarce. A nightly TV habit, for example, can feel relaxing at first but, over time, encroaches on valuable time that could be spent on more meaningful activities. I no longer have a TV, and my life is significantly richer for it. If I want a little chill time with a favorite show, I seek it out online. I watch the Oscars and other major television events at a friend's house. I listen to NPR religiously for my news. After nearly two years this way, I feel as though I've been gifted a great resource of time back in my schedule. Hours do not leak my from daily routine in front of shows that play in the background for company or drain my brain before bed. Better company and a good night's sleep—now, those are great investments!

With whom can you share your abundance?

If you want to be trusted, you must trust. If you want honesty, you must be honest. If you want people to be generous with you, you must be generous with them. It's the law of *karma*—a word that means action. Good actions beget good actions and so on. Moreover, there is no quicker way to feeling the universe's abundance than to give something away to someone who needs it more. When I am feeling particularly low or scarce, I write a thank-you letter to someone else who's done something kind or generous. Volunteering at your local food pantry or simply offering to babysit for a busy friend is a great way to see our own abundance more clearly. Whatever you need, consider giving some of it away. Swami Kripalu put it like this:

> *The universe is exceedingly generous. When a farmer sows one seed, a plant comes forth that produces thousands of seeds. If you desire abundance, be like the farmer and first give up something. Whatever you receive, keep a portion for yourself and share a portion with others. By establishing yourself in the flow of generosity, whatever you give will come back to you manifold.*

4. Remove Obstacles.

When I begin a yoga class with Ganesha mudra, people's eyes light up. Well, first they look at me like I'm a weirdo. *What's a mudra? Who is Ganesha? Save your dogma, lady; just teach me down dog.* (Yoga teachers are accustomed to this kind of thing.) Then, with further explanation, they light up. They sit taller. Their attention sharpens. Eyes brighten around the room, even in lunch hour classes in the Financial District where people arrive preoccupied or sluggish after a busy morning of staring at a computer screen, getting grilled by a client, or schlepping to meetings in uncomfortable shoes. Because for a modern, multitasking yogi, what could be more appealing than the prospect of clearing away some of life's obstacles in mere minutes of sitting still and doing something extremely simple?

It's a long held belief that invoking Ganesha at the start of a yoga class or new stage of any journey removes obstacles from your path and increases the likelihood of success. Which isn't to say that Ganesha obliterates traffic and all of life's travails, but he symbolizes the power of aligning our intentions with the best possible outcome. Call it the Law of Attraction. Call it the Secret. It doesn't matter what you call it, if it works. Focus your mind on the metric of ease, lay the mental groundwork for success, and your path is immediately free of its most daunting and probable obstacle: you. In other words, the inspiration of Ganesha encourages us, above all else, to get out of our own way.

For centuries, Hindus have heartily worshipped this joyful guardian god, who often stands watch in statue form over the threshold of a home. He keeps clear the comings and goings of its inhabitants, bidding them safe journeys and warm returns. Today, yoga practitioners from all religions and cultures are more likely to recognize Ganesha than any other deity. An elephant head is tough to mistake for someone else. He's also popular for having a playful sense of humor. And he has a sweet tooth, so who can't relate to that?

Ganesha says something subtly beautiful about god-energy. It's not just omniscient or all-powerful, as we often think of it. It's also gentle like an elephant, playful like a child, and craves sweets like the rest of us. And, thank goodness, it has a sense of humor—the human equivalent of an obstacle-melting superpower when used wisely. The good news is that we all possess this valuable tool for spiritual sustenance. And therein lies the real gift of Ganesha's symbolism; he makes us think about our role in the creation and destruction of our own obstacles. "The obstacle is the deity," some yogis are fond of saying, rather than its absence. Of course, we'd prefer no traffic, but when traffic arises, that is our truth. It is part of our reality, and how we deal with it—through humor, a shift in perspective, as time to catch up on phone calls (with a hands-free headset of course), or a chance to breathe deeply—either weakens or strengthens our spirits.

It's thrilling when things go our way, but one could make the case that the real yoga practice begins when they don't. We prefer that the elevator doesn't get stuck, it doesn't rain on our wedding day, the economy never tanks, or loved ones never fall ill, but when they do, the spiritual path has not failed us. It's showing us that our devotion to our version of how things should be versus how they are is what causes our suffering. It's giving us a chance to connect to a reserve of strength, empathy, or equanimity we might not otherwise know we had.

The perceived obstacle may just as well create a future blessing. The protracted divorce begets a new love that's a better match. The layoff leads to starting a business, which we might never have had the courage to create otherwise. The untimely death of a loved one leads to the creation of a foundation or research grant to save future generations from a similar fate. Or, maybe we simply remember to count our blessings more often.

Yoga is not useful to a life we *should* live, in a world we wish we had. It is meant for our lives now in this world, as it is. It is not about manufacturing a utopian existence free of setbacks; it's about removing obstacles whenever possible and mastering our own attention and perception when it's not. If we didn't have illusions, we wouldn't need yoga. *Read that again.* The yoga you are doing is not lessened by your daily distractions or stress. It is fueled by it; the distractions and stress are the kerosene for the karmic burning we need to do, to slough off the old and ill-fitting parts of ourselves and become clearer and closer to who we really are.

Whatever happens is as it is and should be—however troubling, painful, or senseless. It cannot be another way. Our practice is to continually show up with courage and grace in the face of any obstacle. When we lack this spiritual strength, we increase the likelihood that when a door of opportunity closes, we spend too much time standing on the stoop cursing rather than look for the proverbial open window. We waste time. We experience more pain than necessary. We cause others pain. We wake the neighbors with all our howling. When we let go of illusion and attachment to how it *should* be according to our own ego, we find the windows more easily. And just as the deities take many forms (of the same god energy), so do obstacles and opportunities. Sometimes, they are one and the same, experienced differently depending on our perspective.

The energy of this deity takes many forms. It's customary to bless a new business owner with a statue or trinket of Ganesha so that her new endeavor is successful. Even before cooking a meal, a prayer can be said to Ganesha to bless its process and completion. But beyond customs in other countries or faiths, the inspiration of Ganesha reminds us that when we begin something new, it helps to set clear intentions to support its success.

Om Work: Meditate and Mind Map

Begin your next meditation with Ganesha mudra

Ganesha's namesake mudra (see pages 160–161) is a great way to focus the mind before meditation or yoga practice or on its own. It also invigorates the body, including the chest, shoulders, biceps, and upper back muscles, which are all in the vicinity of the heart chakra. To weather life's obstacles, it's essential to keep our hearts strong and open. To close this mudra, sit quietly with two hands over your heart and simply listen. The better you get at doing this, the more nimble you will be in body, mind, and spirit when dealing with life's obstacles.

Make a Mind Map

Creating a mind map is one of my all-time favorite ways to invoke a successful journey, project, or life goal. I do it at least twice a year, on New Year's and my birthday (a personal new year), but you can feel free to do it anytime. A mind map provides a powerful and visual way to organize your thoughts around the goals you want to achieve and breaks down how you might attain them. Because how can we expect the universe to deliver our greatest needs and wishes if they remain unknown even to us?

Mind Map Template

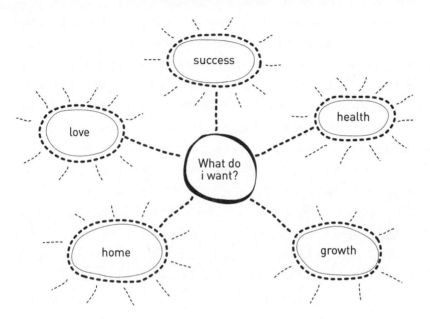

5. Be a Lifelong Student.

Saraswati, the goddess of creativity, writing, music, and education, is my favorite deity. Shocker, right? She represents knowledge, learning, and the joy and importance of being a lifelong student. In India, it's customary for students of all ages to pray to her before exams. She also presides over art, music, and science, and while we don't see her much in yoga, the spirit she embodies supports the yoga principle of *svadhyaya* (self-study), as well as the highest art form any modern yogi practices: life.

There are no elegant poses named for Saraswati, and you're not likely to see her image emblazoned on chic yoga-inspired garb. Trust me, I always try to find her. I would own that garb. She's wont to play second fiddle to Ganesha . . . Scratch that . . . She doesn't play the fiddle. She plays the *veena*, a classical Indian plucked instrument, which resembles a mandolin. Her name means "many rivers," and she's closely associated with water, the essence of life. She wears a white sari and rides a swan.

For creative types, what Saraswati symbolizes isn't merely meaningful; it's how we make meaning of our lives. It's our favorite music, a piece of art we swear was painted by our own soul (provided our soul could paint), or a line of poetry or quote that captures the core of who we are and how we view the world. It makes sense that social media networks and applications such as Facebook, Twitter, Instagram, Tumblr, and Pinterest, which allow people to capture and curate their points of view in words and photos, have become so popular. Likewise with digital music and video-sharing platforms. They might represent new technology, but our instinct for finding and sharing creative expression is timeless.

What was your favorite book as a child? Who read it to you? Name a teacher who had an indelible impact on your education. Which musicians were most popular during your freshman year of high school? If you could decorate your home with a masterpiece by a famous artist, which artist would it be? When you think about it, we're all creative types. We catalogue much of our lives through art, music, education, and culture. What we see. How it makes us feel. What we learn.

Yoga encourages us to keep learning and creating. When we lack inspiration, get stale, experience chronically low energy, or feel depressed, it's because growth and creativity are being stifled. Feeling stifled is serious business; it's the opposite of feeling whole and fully participating in our journey. It's a function of doing someone else's thing rather than your own. "The moment any life, however good, stifles you, you may be sure it isn't your real life," wrote the English poet and essayist Arthur Christopher Benson. All this is to say that yoga is about being real, and being real is born out of respect for your spirit and what makes it come alive. You are whole. You know what is meaningful to you. Conduct your life as a painter paints, as a dancer dances, as an actor takes the stage: follow your passion, nerves be damned!

I have not one, not two, but three small statues of Saraswati in my home, which may sound obsessive, but two of them were gifts transported from India, and it would be rude to get rid of them. So, I look at it this way: some people have ghostwriters to help them write their books; I have Saraswati. You may not identify with her the way I do, but she can still serve as a reminder of the power of creativity and personal artistry. This aspect of who you are, in part, determines the health of your spirit and quality of life.

We know that yoga stretches the capacity of the mind as much (or more) as the body. It teaches us to bear the weight of our emotional lives with greater ease. The key to growth, which is why any of us started doing yoga in the first place (whether we realized it or not), is the ability to learn new things, create new habits, and break old patterns. This phenomenon of "rewiring" your brain is known as neuroplasticity. In her book *Yoga for Emotional Balance*, Bo Forbes, a clinical psychologist, yoga teacher, and personal friend, shares the helpful phrase "Practice makes plastic." Meaning, what we practice becomes ingrained in our neural pathways. When we know better, we can do better. We can treat our bodies more holistically, train our minds to be more present, and invite our spirits to take the lead more often.

Saraswati, as a symbol of learning, reminds us to keep things that inspire us at the forefront of our lives. Her energy is in our favorite music, daydreams, and doodled drawings; the fresh pages of a new journal, a business brainstorm, or conflict resolution that feels like a perfect plot twist in a great novel: unexpected yet inevitable. *I've got it!* we say, in an epiphanic moment. Yet, the foundation was there all along. Finally, creative juices flow. The muse arrives. Our om thing is in the house. Saraswati bids us never to stop learning. Not to pack away our childhood instruments in the attic to gather dust if they still bring us joy. She inspires us to register for the cooking or martial arts class we resolved to take last New Year's (and several years before that), and choose job opportunities that, above all, foster growth. A different sort of powerful female figure and by certain standards a modern goddess of Silicon Valley, Facebook COO Sheryl Sandberg, writes in her book *Lean In* that the single most important metric for making career decisions is potential for growth. It's the basis upon which she chose to work at Google in its earliest days and, later, as COO of Facebook when plenty of other companies were offering her coveted CEO roles. About this, she quips, "At first, people questioned why I would take a 'lower level' job working for a twenty-three-year-old. No one asks me that anymore."

We've all had the experience of working at a job that doesn't inspire us. I once did a stint as the director of marketing at a high-profile commercial real estate company in Boston. I made a handsome salary. I worked humane hours, especially in comparison to my incessant yoga teaching and magazine-life schedules. I'd look up at 5:05 to notice that most of my colleagues were gone for the night. The people were kind. The environment was healthy. The CEO trusted me implicitly. He was smart and impeccable. I took the job because I wanted to learn from him and someday develop the pluck to start my own business. Overnight, I was the most senior-ranking woman in the company. And, yet, many evenings I would arrive home, put my forehead against the cool glass of my kitchen table, and sob my face off. I was literally bored to tears. My skills outmatched my duties, especially in a slowing economy, and I was sad with the lack of work or opportunities for growth among peers who challenged me. My spirit was shriveling. I could feel it.

It can feel selfish or self-indulgent to devote resources toward the health of our spirit, especially in a culture of scarcity such as ours or at the cost of a salary or title for which we've worked hard. However, the most costly mistake we can make in life and business is *not* listening to our spirits, to sell our souls, you could say. Ignoring our personal growth, heart's desire, or spiritual yearning is the quickest and most direct route to feeling, well, *dispirited*. When we overlook the spirit of creativity, learning, and growth—the essence of Saraswati—we fracture and distance ourselves from the source of what makes us most luminous and successful.

Instead of viewing spiritual work as separate from our physical or financial health, we must remember that the world *needs* strong spirits. To have a fulfilling life, you must be true to your spirit. You must create and grow. Moreover, when your spirit is at its strongest, it creates the most rewarding opportunities. Its currency is different in terms of dollars and cents, but it makes life richer.

Here are a few ways to reignite creative inspiration and sustain spirit through the energy associated with Saraswati (e.g., art, music, education, and continuing development).

Om Work: Live Artfully

Practice Pratyhara

Have you ever struggled to come up with a creative idea or resolve a nagging problem only to have your eureka moment in the shower? It happens to me all the time. So much so that when I worked in media I would joke in meetings that I'd have the fresh tagline of copy or best solution to a client problem the next day. I'd admit that the answer would inevitably be coming to me in the shower. I started to wonder if I should get a waterproof computer. Think of how productive I'd be! Until quickly realizing that the lack of stimulus and change of scenery are precisely why I had my best ideas in the shower. Time to unplug is paramount for the creative process; the mind needs space and quiet to breathe and find new courses of action. Remember your modern-day practices of pratyhara: turn off all screens, remove your earbuds, nix the TV for the night (or the week or forever), and plug inward. The boldest and brightest ideas and epiphanies will come when you are quiet enough to hear their arrival.

Go Back to School

Learning new things is one of the best ways to reinvigorate the mind and lift the spirit. If you're feeling stale or uninspired, perhaps it's time to sign up for a class, go back to school, or seek continuing education opportunities within your career or area of passion. Alternatively, teaching others is another surefire way to light your own creative fire, even if it's as small as a child's shoelace with its bunny rabbit running around the hole or helping a parent learn a new form of technology. My greatest inspirations for this book often came from explaining an idea or philosophical concept to students. Continually and actively participating in the learning process from both sides is one of our most renewable and reliable forms of inspiration and creativity.

Learn a New Yoga Style

While working as a member of the teaching staff on a yoga teacher-training retreat—typically full of starry-eyed young yogis—I met a student named Stephanie who was already burned out upon arrival. Hailing from New York City, the first (and last) open smoker I'd ever seen on a yoga retreat, Stephanie was brash and more vocal than most yoga teachers allowed themselves to be at the time. "Sometimes, I want to punch yoga in face," she confessed. In my early twenties and still very yoga starry-eyed myself, I was aghast. However, I would soon learn how severe yoga burnout, like any other form of burnout, could be. Certainly it's not yoga's fault, but it's up to us to continually refill our wellspring of inspiration. Whether you tire of teaching yoga or practicing it, the answer is the same: take a step back, stop plowing ahead, and do something that lights up your inspiration (preferably not a cigarette). A new yoga style, studio, or teacher can work wonders for our creative experiences on and off the mat. Or, spend some time off the mat altogether.

Visit with Nature

Who knows creativity and growth better than Mother Nature? There's a reason people talk about finding inspiration or God, or both really, on mountaintops. The air is clearer up there. Our egos step aside. The elements do not yield to meet our self-serving needs. No one can grease the palm of a rainstorm to buy it off. For this reason and many others, nature is the ultimate equalizer and muse. It resets our self-involvement and forces us to think broader, breathe bigger, and feel deeper. We let go and *let in*. You don't have to travel far or long, and if it's too cold or late at night to sit on a park bench and feed the ducks or take a walk along the beach, then keeping houseplants or watching the sunset will do in a pinch. Heck, even watching a surf documentary will do. Watch the expert at work. Contemplate how nature does her thing. Then, you can return to doing yours with a fresh perspective.

Live an Artful Life

Knowing our strengths is paramount to doing our om thing—and knowing our weaknesses. Of these, some of mine include letting go, setting boundaries, reading maps (not of the mind map variety), and singing. (There are plenty more.) The singing is spectacularly bad. Which might be why I have such a deep appreciation for live music. In particular, I love the collective spirit a live show creates. If our most primal need as humans is to connect, music is so often the glue. Sustain your spirit and the collective spirit of creativity by supporting the arts. Go to a concert. Visit a museum. Attend an art opening. Marvel at a dance performance. You don't have to see a legendary rock show at Madison Square Garden or a professional ballet company's performance to let creativity move you. Simply bask in the human experience conveyed through different mediums and honor its spirit in yourself and others. You don't have to be an artist to live an artful life or carry a tune to give voice to inspiration. I love the way Helena Bonham Carter describes this idea: "I think everything in life is art. What you do, how you dress, the way you love someone, and how you talk. Your smile and your personality. What you believe in, and all your dreams. The way you drink your tea. How you decorate your home. Or party. Your grocery list. The food you make. How your writing looks. And the way you feel."

6. Put Your Foot Down

Perhaps all the dragons in our lives are princesses who are only waiting to see us act, just once, with beauty and courage. Perhaps everything that frightens us is, in its deepest essence, something helpless that wants our love.

—RAINER MARIA RILKE, *LETTERS TO A YOUNG POET*

Without exposure to the gods and goddesses of Hinduism, it might seem counterintuitive, disturbing, or depraved that there would be a goddess like Kali who resides in a cremation ground, painted with blue cremation ashes, and wielding a sword dripping in blood. She stands with one foot on the chest of her husband, Shiva. In her hand, she holds a decapitated head, a garland of human skulls around her neck, all the while sticking out her tongue in a wild, fierce expression. To put it bluntly: Kali is fricking terrifying. This may cause you to wonder, what, if anything, does this goddess of raging power and wrath have to do with the peaceful practice of yoga?

Before we sort through all that, let's first clarify why Hindus worship Kali. Her devotees do not see her as threatening nor do they hope to emulate her wrath and violence. Rather, they see her as a protective and nurturing mother figure, roaring and rearing only in the direction of evil and illusion. If there's a bully stuffing a kid in a locker somewhere or dictator oppressing a group of people, Kali is the deity we wish we could send in to regulate. That's the image she conjures. She also reminds us of life's cyclical nature; from any-thing destroyed something beautiful and new can emerge. Her role is that of the redeemer. Most of all, her job is to destroy what holds us back from the truth. She slays illusion, levels b.s., and scares away evil.

For modern yogis, Kali demonstrates that emotions like anger and rage are not bad or unyogic. They are human. It's what we do with them that define us. Sometimes we must figuratively put our foot down, as she literally does on Shiva's chest. We must stick out our tongues to scare a would-be predator or roar viciously in the di-rection of something that threatens our cubs. A modern yogi man-tra I've heard circulating lately captures this sentiment perfectly: *Do no harm, but take no shit.* I don't know where to attribute this gem, but it is the lesson of Kali, who is also an incarnation of the warrior goddess Durga. Her symbolism for us is that we must not confuse being a peaceful yogi with being a pushover. Instead, we must stand up for ourselves when necessary, like the ahimsa par-able of the snake, and also be brave enough to walk onto the scary grounds of our own dark emotions and take action. The most fear-less warriors are the ones who can shine a light on their own dark-ness. Because when we deny or hide our dark sides, they find us all the same. The modern yoga community unfortunately offers ample examples of this. How often have exalted gurus revealed them-selves to be dishonest, exploitative, or abusive, as if their glowing façade wouldn't eventually crumble? The message seems simple: address your shadowy side or it will overtake you.

The archetype of Kali reminds us that the precursor to healing and transformation is sometimes anger. Abraham Lincoln, Ma-hatma Gandhi, Martin Luther King Jr., and Nelson Mandela all got angry at the inequality and injustice around them. They may have wanted to rage at cowardice and complacency, as if brandish-ing swords, but they fought and led with love instead. They transformed historical periods of darkness into legacies of light for us to follow.

The beautiful postures we do are yoga, but so is the reckoning of our lives, from feelings into action. It's not about ignoring negative emotions or events to be more virtuous, peaceful, or attractive. Most of us learn the hard way that people pleasing has its limits, if not perils. Having an unpolished and imposing spiritual symbol like Kali reminds yogis to be fierce and have faith that protection can come to us in the most unlikely, and even unpleasant, places and forms.

The darkest periods of humanity often cause people to question the existence of God. Why would God allow this tragedy? If there is a God, he/she can't be here today, in this rubble, devastation, or depravity. *No God would let this happen.* The principle of Kali assures us that God doesn't sleep. He or she is nearby and deep within, so often revealing—in our darkest moments—our most illuminating strength of ourselves and those around us. A fierce and protective love can rise from anything: the ash, rubble, breakup, or a part of ourselves that needs to be destroyed so that another can flourish.

Om Work: Be Fierce

Break or Burn Something

What's the matter? You look skeptical. You look like I've just told you to do something outlandishly unyogic, like eat gluten or wear high heels. The thing about burning or breaking things is that it's cathartic. It feels fierce. It feels unquestionably Kali. It helps us handle the baggage we all carry of being ourselves, and, frankly, that is yoga. "Yoga is the practice of tolerating the consequences of being yourself," the *Bhagavad Gita* says. The key is to be discerning about what you're breaking or burning, and save the activity for special occasions. I hear chopping wood is exhilarating. In my city life, I like to stomp the small sheets of ice that form over puddles in the winter. Burning things (appropriate things, in fire-safe environments) is also oddly fulfilling. I often incorporate fire as a ritual element at the end of a teacher-training program, on the final night of a yoga retreat, or to conclude one of my off-the-mat courses. Few things feel as good and redemptive as writing down the name of the person, feeling, or bad habit that's holding you back, crumpling it up, tossing it into a bonfire or kitchen sink, and watching it go up in flames.

Get Fierce About Fitness

I've been candid about how modern yoga overprioritizes its fitness aspect over all else. Personally, I don't enjoy when yoga is my sole form of fitness, and I observe what it does to my students on their mats when they do this, as well. If your yoga mat is also your only realm for working out, it can all too easily become a place for rushing, competing, obligation, overexertion, and injury. Moreover, certain emotions are better metabolized off the mat, especially anger, envy, and rage. For this reason, there are times when the path to inner peace may come by way of getting off the mat and into a more ferocious form of fitness, such as running, boxing, or interval training. Your mat is a sacred space, but damn, it feels good to moonlight in environments that welcome some swagger. It also provides a healthy balance for mind and body (which thrives on a combination of strength, flexibility, and cardiovascular training).

Talk Back to That Voice

You know the dark voice in your head? The one who convinces you that you're not good enough, smart enough, or strong enough to live your truth? It keeps us in destructive relationships, hooked to unhealthy habits, and scared of taking chances. It convinces us this is as good as it gets. Don't dream any bigger, you'll only be disappointed. The devil you know is better than the one you don't. Sure. Fine. There's an inkling of truth to that. But why don't we ever hear the opposite? *Look out—it just might work out better than you could possibly imagine.* After spending years with some very scared and unhealthy voices, I finally learned that they don't just go away. They don't pack up and leave politely. Voices of fear, self-doubt, and sabotage are vicious and unrelenting . . . *until* the day you talk back to them. My friend Abby taught me this. She's an English teacher who specializes in Toni Morrison and Leo Tolstoy, which you might find a delightful juxtaposition to the choice words she shared with me. We were sitting on her deck one day, sharing a bowl of cherries, when she declared, "You need to talk back to that voice and say: Fuck YOU." It was stern advice, but it was dead-on. Identify the scared, insecure, sometimes evil, always ego-driven voices and sic your inner Kali on them.

7. Leap!

We have to continually be jumping off cliffs and developing our wings on the way down.

—Kurt Vonnegut

Kurt Vonnegut's words are another blast of a trumpet for me. So, they belong in my personal bible. They get me closer to my om thing. They also remind me of the monkey god, Hanuman, who famously leapt through the forest in the *Ramayana* to help his friend Rama look for his wife, Sita, who had been abducted. From this harrowing and epic tale, Hanumanasana, known in yoga classes as a split, gets its name, since our legs resemble the *grand jeté* shape of the monkey god's as he leapt through the Sri Lankan forest from tree to tree.

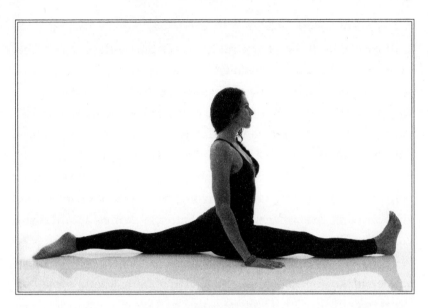

Hanumanasana
(Split)

Hanuman represents deep, abiding devotion and great physical strength. He is a symbol of courage, as well as friendship, and his existence in yoga philosophy is inextricably linked to his best friend, Rama. He is also known for being an impeccable student and immune to fatigue. His devotion was said to fuel his superhuman strength, a deep sense of purpose powering him through the universe. A favorite story of mine is when Hanuman was once sent to retrieve a medicinal herb from the mountainside for a sick friend. When he arrived, he couldn't remember how to identify which herb he needed. Not wanting to let down his friend, he decided, instead, to carry the whole mountain back with him, which would be like the present-day equivalent of having a terrible cold and asking your sweetheart to go to CVS for you. Once there, your sweetheart isn't sure which medicine you need, so he or she brings back the whole dang pharmacy. Now that's love.

Hanuman's myth also says he traversed the sky backward to keep pace with the sun since his guru was Surya, the sun god (for whom sun salutations are named). If he wanted to learn the lessons Surya had to teach, Hanuman needed an indefatigable spirit. To know a sliver of Hanuman's story is to know that he is devoted, strong, and true. Nothing stops him. Nothing fatigues him. In his faith, he finds boundless energy and a sense of safety. He reminds us that we're more likely to leap when we believe in who's jumping (ourselves!). And living a life of purpose, with a devotion to others, gives us a safety net when we leap. Or better yet, wings, according to Vonnegut.

Doing a full split in yoga class is wonderful, but it pales in comparison to the importance of taking leaps of faith, whether small or large, in daily life. What cultivates this courage of spirit is not flexible hamstrings, it's faith in ourselves and/or a higher power. We learn to release our need to know and control what comes next. We loosen our grasp of how it *should* be. We embrace what is. Instead of seeing the unknown as terrifying, we are more willing to see it as full of possibility. We let go. Rather than leaping away from life, we leap toward it.

"The task of life is to face sacred moments," wrote rabbi and Jewish theologian Abraham Joshua Heschel, which implies that sacred moments come in all forms, even the ordinary or scary. We learn this and forget it continuously. We grow small or scared again, and we need to be reminded (again) of our power and purpose. That's what yoga is for. That's what Hanuman is for or your own version of his lessons. Being devoted to your own spirit and path helps you to be your bravest self. Life is a process of remembering not only to leap into uncertainty but also to trust that your wings will appear each time you do. No matter who you are, your life is comprised of many leaps each day—small and large—to try something new, stand up for something in which you believe, take the plunge into a new industry, fall in love, start a business, or launch yourself toward a faith that someone or something will catch you on the other side. Here are some ways to make sure you are ready for your next leap.

Om Work: Take a Leap

Be Stronger than Your Fears

People pray to Hanuman for strength. He is a soldier god, one who inspires courage. Whether your courageous leap is physical or not, having a strong, healthy body will give you added energy and stamina for your journey. Try incorporating bursts of strength into your yoga or exercise routine. For example, try doing longer holds of standing poses, like Warriors I and II, Utkatasana (Chair Pose), or a variation of Chair Pose done against a wall, squeezing a block between your inner thighs. Practice remaining calm and relaxed as your body quivers or fatigues. A one-minute hold is challenging for most people and a great, simple dose of strength for your body's largest muscle groups: glutes and thighs. Other options might include running uphill or lifting weights. Remember, if Hanuman can carry a mountain, you can climb one of your own. As you become physically stronger, encourage your own lionhearted strength with the mantra: *I am stronger than my fears.*

Leap with a Friend

When partnerships—professional, personal, or romantic—align with our highest Self and are acts of loyalty and devotion, we never leap alone. This feeling has a ripple effect through everything we do. It strengthens and energizes us. It gives us the power to take greater and farther leaps in all areas of life. I want you to know this feeling is real and possible, and my greatest wish is that your om thing helps you find and foster partnerships that make you feel unstoppable.

Play a Power Anthem

The Hanuman Chalisa is a traditional chant sung for strength and courage. Feel free to download a version and use it, or find your own song, something that makes you feel invincible. "Eye of the Tiger." "We Will Rock You." "Respect." "Roar" . . . Let yourself be puffed up by the bravado of Jay-Z or inspired by the originality of Lady Gaga. Get thee a power anthem, and pump it loud whenever you need a launching pad for your next big leap.

8. Find Your Flow.

From birth, we each have our own rhythm. We're introverts or extroverts, early birds or night owls. We plod, then pounce, or pounce, then plod. We feed off the energy of a group or cherish solitude. Our ideas come like fireworks, popping off brighter and louder than the next. Or, we mull things over, needing time to live with a thought before trying it out in the world. We cannonball. We dip a toe. We need someone to light a fire under us. *Eff that, I am the fire.* We meditate first thing. We need a cup of coffee before conversation is feasible. We're sprinters; we're marathoners. We crave a cozy couch, plush throw blankets, and a rainy day. We keep a notepad by the bed in case something important comes to us in the middle of the night. We're of the strong, scientifically backed opinion that few things are as important as sleep. We take a while to warm up. We're open books. *What do you want to know?* Each of us is a unique combination of energy and potential.

As we age, our internal rhythm shifts. We awake earlier when a newborn cries or big prospective client meeting is scheduled. We burn the midnight oil when dharma calls. But, ultimately, we have a default setting. We have preferences and a natural pace. Our mothers might attest that we were this way even as babies. A friend of mine says that all three of her children exhibited key aspects of their personalities in the delivery room: watchful, fiery, and easygoing. In Ayurveda, the traditional system of healing that aligns with yoga philosophy and enhances yoga practice, this internal rhythm and matrix of our own nature is called our *prakruti*, which combines three primary components, known as *doshas*. Ayurveda is a comprehensive field, but the most basic principle is that all of us are comprised of all the elements: earth, water, fire, air, and space (also known as ether). When we have too much of one and not enough of others, we're prone to imbalance or illness. We can literally be too fired up or airy, for example. Typically capable and focused, I can be a total airhead when my life is out of balance. In response, I move faster. I try to do more, and eventually, my mind can't keep up. It brings to mind the time, while on deadline to complete this book, that my car was stolen.

Initially, I thought it was towed. Except no tow lots in the City of Boston could find my car, nor could the police. Over the phone, a BPD officer's voice, as if from central casting for a role in a Mark Wahlberg film, told me to report it stolen.

"I'm sorry ma'am, but we don't have yah cah."

I cried. Until I realized my car wasn't towed or stolen. I just forgot where I parked it. A mind can only handle so much.

In my earlier incarnations as a yogi, I may have had a sinking suspicion I wasn't a "real yogi." Too far from Zen, too close to Crazy. Now I know I'm human (and I parked my car near the coffee shop not the Thai restaurant). Yoga is a practice, and learning to find your way back to balance is part of the deal. A willingness to practice and be present is all that's required to be a real yogi. Through yoga, we learn to observe and manage our energy and become more aware of the flow of energy all around us. We amplify the work of our bodies by economizing the energy of our spirit. And even when we're convinced our highest self has been towed elsewhere, our rhythm completely out of sync with the universe, yoga helps us find it again. It's also why understanding the subtle body is so important to self-care.

You'll recall that Shiva is the creator and destroyer of the universe, like a spiritual Big Bang or version of Shakira that dances and shakes the cosmos into motion. His incarnation of Nataraja, which means

Lord of the Dance, is the inspiration for one of the most popular asanas that we do, Dancer's Pose (Natarajasana, page 107). Nataraja's dance both orders the world and creates its chaos, since the natural rhythm of life is one of flux and change. Images of Nataraja dancing in a ring of fire are prominent in yoga studios. You've probably seen many without realizing it.

So, what does it mean when *you* do Dancer's Pose? Whatever you want it to mean, of course! We all dance to the beat of our own proverbial drum. It can be just a test of balancing on one foot, with a decent quadriceps stretch and a fun backbend. Or, you might like to know that your body language nods to the tradition of yoga in this pose. It says something about life. That all its elements are within you, as well as around you. It says that the skill is to be in the moment, as it is, even when it feels chaotic or terrifying, as though dancing in a ring of fire. The deity, made into a standing backbend on one leg, reminds us that we have our own rhythm, and we belong to a greater rhythm and flow of life, which vibrates and pulses endlessly. Even when standing impeccably still, trillions of cells within our bodies are moving, changing, dying, and rejuvenating. They restore themselves completely every seven years, a constant tango of destruction and creation. We dance with change even when seemingly standing still.

My boyfriend once told me that Dancer's Pose was one of his favorites.

"Why?" I asked.

"I don't know; it feels like I'm doing yoga," he said simply.

Om Work: Find Your Rhythm

Determine your dosha.

Learn your dosha with a simple Ayurvedic chart like the one provided on page 235, to better understand and honor your personal constitution and natural rhythm.

In each chart category, choose the characteristic that fits you most, dating as far back as you remember. You are trying to determine the "default setting" with which you were born. Once you determine your dosha, you can learn more about keeping it balanced with yoga and Ayurveda.

How to Determine Your Dosha

	VATA	PITTA	KAPHA
BODY FRAME	Thin, sinewy, tall or short.	Medium build.	Larger frame.
WEIGHT	Hard to gain, easy to lose.	Easy to gain, easy to lose.	Easy to gain, hard to lose.
SKIN	Cold, dark undertones, tans easily.	Warm, light, sunburns or flushes easily.	Cool, fair, oily, thick.
HAIR	Dry, frizzy, thin.	Straight, fine, prone to loss or premature graying.	Thick, wavy, lustrous.
EYES	Small, active, brown or black.	Green, hazel, almond-shaped.	Big, calm, blue.
APPETITE	Fluctuates.	Intense.	Consistent.
SWEAT	Glistens.	Buckets.	Perspires.
TEMPERAMENT	Fearful, indecisive, nervous, perceptive.	Angry, intelligent, arrogant, successful.	Greedy, calm, stable, stubborn.
MEMORY	Learns quickly, forgets quickly.	Learns quickly, forgets slowly.	Learns slowly, forgets slowly.
SPEECH	Erratic, talkative.	Articulate, decisive.	Slow, cautious.
CLIMATE	Dislikes cold, dry.	Dislikes heat and humidity.	Dislikes humidity.
ACTIVITY	Restless and active.	Competitive and fierce.	Calm and leisurely.
ROUTINES	Dislikes routine.	Likes planning and organizing.	Works well with routine.

Dance.

Dancing lifts the spirit. It makes life's burdens less daunting. It sloughs off grouchiness before it has a chance to settle and harden like plaster.

Read this quote by legendary dancer Martha Graham.

"I believe that we learn by practice. Whether it means to learn to dance by practicing dancing or to learn to live by practicing living, the principles are the same. In each, it is the performance of a dedicated precise set of acts, physical or intellectual, from which comes the shape of achievement, a sense of one's being, a satisfaction of spirit. One becomes, in some area, an athlete of God. Practice means to perform, over and over again in the face of all obstacles, some act of vision, of faith, of desire. Practice is a means of inviting the perfection desired."

9. Build a sangha.

Large corporations have boards of directors. Small start-ups have advisory boards. The President has a cabinet. A race car driver has a pit crew. Yoga encourages us to have something similar, a spiritual board of directors if you will.

The yoga equivalent is called a *sangha.** It's a spiritual community of people whom you trust, who inspire you, whose wisdom you can draw upon because they've been there. You may find yours at a yoga studio, meditation center, on a sports team, at an artists' collective, by joining a book club, or in an online forum. Or, you can assemble your own, collecting friends and sages from various corners of your life and letting them share your journey and weigh in when life weighs you down. You can do this in person, or, through the advent of technology, via phone, email, or Skype, to name a few ways to keep in touch. "No man is an island," wrote John Donne. Ditto the modern yogi. After all, the word "yoga" means *to connect.*

Connection and a sense of community are one of humankind's most primal needs. People crave the feeling of being part of a collective greater than themselves. We form tribes, join clubs, and congre-

....

* *Sangha* is the term used in Buddhism. In Sanskrit, the same concept is called *sat-sang.* I use sangha because I see it more often in the yoga community, which is often cross-pollinated by Buddhism, and I sustain my spiritual life with many aspects of Buddhist philosophy.

gate. It's the *ujjayi* breath of a yoga class or hearty vibration of many voices chanting *om*. One could argue that the rise in yoga's popularity is, in part, an answer to a decline in the prevalence of religious communities. A yoga community can fulfill a spiritual need without involving religious beliefs or doctrine or supplement the community you create for yourself elsewhere (religious or otherwise).

Ancient yoga wisdom is full of community. The deities, discussed here as symbols of our own spiritual journeys rather than objects of worship, often travel in packs. Like celebrities, each one has an entourage, including a consort (lover), parents, companions, and a *vahana* or vehicle by which they travel (e.g,. Lakshmi in the lotus flower; Saraswati on a swan; Ganesha, the elephant god, with a tiny mouse, of all things). Roots of the practice in India evolved from intimate relationships between a guru and student to a guru and ashram full of students. Eventually, Westerners were allowed into these ashrams, and yoga proliferated exponentially. Today's definition of doing yoga is inextricably linked to where we do it and with whom.

But more than anything, good people are good for your spirit. Off the mat, we create support systems of people who ground us, lift us, and infuse our lives with inspiration and creativity. When we lean on these friends, mentors, and personal champions, we feel buoyed by their wisdom or love. We're happier, more productive, held by their experience and support. They don't have to be yogis at all, but their overall effect on our lives is one of greater balance. When we alienate ourselves from them, for any number of reasons, we can feel lonely or stuck. The suggestion, therefore, is not merely to have a network of people whom you trust but to entrust them *before* you are stuck and depleted of spiritual sustenance. Share a business idea when it's only a glimmer, voice fear before it swallows you whole, or mention a problem before it snowballs into a catastrophe. Paramount to cultivating and maintaining a strong support system is knowing who is best qualified and most excited about helping you and in which areas of your life. For example, I wouldn't suggest bringing your troubles in the boudoir to your career mentor.

Just as the three supreme gods, Brahma, Visnu, and Shiva, preside over all areas of the universe—its creation, preservation, and destruction—you likely have primary pillars of support and sources of inspiration in your sangha. These select people are your life's brightest and most precious gems, to whom you can go with anything. They might include your BFF, partner, a parent, sibling, or therapist. Meanwhile, like specialist deities who preside over a specific area of the universe, you also have friends, colleagues, and confidantes whom you most trust with a special role in your life. Lakshmi for success. Saraswati for knowledge. Kali for being a badass. Your tough-love friend, guardian angel, and sounding board. Your comic relief. Your ambassador of cool.

Members of your sangha go by many names: friends, mentors, sages, spiritual guides, personal champions, and heroes, to name a few. But to some degree, they're all sages who have something important to teach. Yoga tradition is filled with sages. Seven of whom make up the *saptarishi*, a group of teachers first mentioned in the earliest Vedic texts including the Upanishads.

Without realizing it, you've performed or marveled at one or more poses that pay homage to an ancient sage of yoga. They are often some of the most challenging poses (frequently in the arm-balance family), since the sages were known for having a lot of *tapas*, the disciplinary, purifying fire we talked about in the first section. You'll recall it's one of the *niyamas* (attitudes toward the self). Particularly visible poses today that are named for sages include but are not limited to Astavakrasana, Galavasana, Vasisthasana, and Visvamitrasana.

Of these, the sage Astavakra has a particularly moving story. As legend has it, Astavakra was born crippled, his body bent in eight places. For this reason, the pose is translated as Eight-Angle Pose (page 102). Astavakra's body was so compromised he could barely stand up, let alone do asana. Yet, he showed an early affinity for yoga philosophy and knack for understanding the wisdom of the Vedas. Even from the womb, he would correct his father for mispronouncing Sanskrit words. His father did not find this amusing, and he would curse the unborn child, his ire causing the boy's body to warp and recoil in eight different places. After his birth and once he got older, Astavakra went to visit a guru who was teaching a class of yogis, who immediately began to laugh at him. How could he study yoga when he couldn't even stand, they mocked! What kind of yogi looked the way he did?

"You're not yogis," Astavakra calmly replied. "You're shoemakers."

This only made the exclusive and judgmental yogis laugh harder, until Astavakra explained himself. "If you think that my body is my identity, this skin in which I live is all there is of me, you might as well make shoes out of it."

At this point, the guru realized he had made a terrible error, allowing his students to evaluate yoga achievement on the basis of appearances. He then showed great deference to Astavakra and invited him to teach the group.

How ironic that we still get so wrapped up in the appearances of yoga and overidentification with the physical body. We focus on what poses like Astavakrasana look like, often forgetting that there's deeper wisdom awaiting us beneath the surface. Next time you attempt this pose or another hotshot arm balance or inversion, go for it with every fiber of your being. Use your tapas, like the sages did. Strengthen your body and discipline your mind with the focus these efforts require, but remember that each pose has a spirit, too. With practice, we bring this spirit to the surface and see it in others more readily, no matter what the outside looks like.

Like Astavakra revealing his wisdom to the yogis, your spiritual board of advisors will reveal itself to you over time. Maybe they'll come in the form of yogis who plan vegan potlucks and go on retreats together. Maybe they won't resemble yogis at all but, instead, carry their practice inwardly. All the same, they'll make you feel more like yourself. They'll help you see clearly. They'll teach you what they know. When we bow to these people, we lift ourselves.

Om Work: Find a Tribe

Elect Your Board of Directors

People love to know how important they are to you. It puffs them up, like getting the best classroom job in grammar school. *Look at me, guys, I get to clap the erasers! I am the chosen one who gets to make noise and exhilarating clouds of chalk in the air.* Nothing makes any of us feel more alive than having a sense of purpose, and nowhere is God's grace more present than when people support each other. By confiding in your people and identifying and appreciating their special role in your life, you strengthen all the spirits involved: yours, theirs, and the collective one contained in your bond.

Number for yourself those most protective of and empowering to your spiritual life, then tell someone that they are your hero, mentor, personal champion, or ambassador of hip (this is what I call my graphic designer, Matt), and watch that person rise to the occasion. Watch the cluster of blessings around you multiply. Watch your own spirit puff up a little, with a very important job to do.

Meet Regularly

"Meeting regularly" for the modern yogi is highly subjective. We might see a mentor daily at the office and meet a hero once in a lifetime. We might talk to our greatest personal champion each night before drifting off to sleep or once a month (whenever one of us prevails at phone tag). What's important is that we set a regular intention to plug into these sources of energy and support and—as the law of karma insists—return the favor, too.

Welcome Spiritual Guidance

It's customary in many spiritual practices, including yoga, to create small altars for gods, gurus, or guides who have passed on to the other side and spend time in ritual with them. In Hindu culture and yoga tradition, these are called *pujas*. They can be grounding and centering places for our spirits to sit quietly, commune with a higher power, pray, talk, meditate, cry, chant, think, not think . . . whatever is needed as an ablution of the heart that day. Especially for the urban-dwelling yogi, a small altar can offer sacred space even when there isn't much actual space to be had.

I encourage you to create a physical space that aligns with the things you want to hold space for in your soul. The book *Care of the Soul* by Thomas Moore offers many beautiful examples of this idea. It might be as simple as keeping a photo of one of your heroes at your desk, dedicating a nook of your bookshelf to an inspiration, or creating a serene space in your home to do yoga without the glare of a nearby computer or eyesore of dirty laundry. It might need to be on the kitchen floor because that surface is best for your mat and most clear of furniture and other obstructions (this was the case for me for a couple years), but you can still lovingly light a candle and display meaningful objects nearby to signal your openness for spiritual guidance while you practice. A photo of a faraway friend or late relative, shell from a favorite beach where you always feel calm and whole, mala beads from a retreat that changed you, or a mantra written on a piece of paper—anything can transform the place where you make oatmeal into a mini sanctuary. If it opens and soothes your heart or mind or both, that's all the guidance you need.

Bow Deeply

Even the most selfless and optimistic among us can feel like Debbie Downer sometimes, griping more than usual and leaning heavily on our inner circles. Luckily, sangha members worth their salt know we will snap out of it, and, eventually, we do. When this happens, it's not only important to thank your people but to share happier news in the days ahead. I think of this as the repaying of an emotional loan.

Share a joyous photo with your new love after the hellacious breakup, new dog after the tearful good-bye of your former canine friend, or standing outside your new office after too many scary and scarce months of unemployment. Send the blog post you wrote about an ordinary but magical moment. Remember to mark not only the hardships with which you needed help but the contentment and clarity your sangha helped you create. I've been known to send my therapist thank-you notes months or years after the last time I've seen her. It must be odd to listen to all that crying, offer patient counsel, put someone's pieces together again, and then hear nothing more. If the yoga path is about becoming whole, part of the yoga practice for you might include recognizing the people who were, at times, your glue. Not to mention there is a beautiful multiplier effect. To summarize artist, writer, and poet Khalil Gibran, sorrow shared is cut in half. Joy shared doubles.

> *"Do the work; stay out of the misery."*
> —MAHARISHI MAHESH YOGI

You Get Good at What You Practice

Maybe it's because of the prevalence of social media today, with anyone able to amplify their grievances at any time, or too much reality TV, but it seems as though we're getting more comfortable talking about how *dispirited* we are. There's a protracted war in one corner of the globe and lots of teetering on the brink in others, an unwieldy economy, a pervasive loneliness that Likes and Friends cannot soothe. No one needs help enumerating our spiritual maladies, whether personal or collective.

On the other hand, we're less comfortable talking about the presence of spirit. How to make our own feel whole, how to sleep better at night, how to feel as though our life is meaningful, not happening by accident or hurtling by too fast. If we can talk about feeling dispirited so easily, why can't we talk about becoming full of spirit? I don't have the answer, but it probably includes something about it being difficult and potentially hokey. In yoga circles, it includes debates that move from just wanting a good workout to ancient tradition and back again. Everywhere else, whenever the conversation about spirit bumps up against religion and God, people get uncomfortable and often give up. Why pray if we don't know whom we're talking to? Why honor yoga's tradition if we're not Hindu? Why bother with anything else if our lives are too full and fast-moving already?

I can't pretend to have the answers to all of these questions or any of them, but I do know that having a relationship with your spirit is better than not having one, feeling propelled by purpose generally makes people happier and healthier, and feeling a source of light within and around you brightens every aspect of life. I don't think you have to be religious to pray. I don't think you have to sacrifice the fitness of yoga to respect its tradition. I do think respecting yoga's tradition is imperative to calling what we're doing *yoga*.

The following prayer is one that I frequently share with my students. It is not limited to any particular faith or spiritual practice, and I think you'll see many of the universal truths that unite both shining through. It was given to me by my friend Jennelle, the runner who towed me up Heartbreak Hill in the dead of winter. My hope is that next time your spirit needs to be pulled through something difficult or you want to pray but don't know how to start talking, you can use this or piece together another prayer or practice, on your mat or off, to create your om thing.

Radiant Prayer

The supreme prayer of my heart . . . is not to be rich, famous, powerful, or too good, but to be radiant. I desire to radiate health, calm courage, cheerfulness, and good will. I wish to live without hate, whim, jealousy, envy, or fear. I wish to be simple, honest, frank, natural, clean in mind and clean in body, unaffected, ready to say I do not know if so it be, to meet all men and women on an absolute equality, to face any obstacle and meet every difficulty unabashed and unafraid. I wish others to live their lives, too, up to their fullest and best. To that end, I pray that I may never meddle, interfere, dictate, give advice that is not wanted, or assist when my services are not needed. If I can help people, I will do it, by giving them a chance to help themselves; and if I can uplift or inspire, let it be by example, rather than by injunction and dictation. That is to say, I desire to be radiant, to radiate life.

—ELBERT HUBBARD

CHAPTER 11

Love

*"In the end only three things matter: how well we have lived, how
well we have loved, and how well we have learned to let go."*
—JACK KORNFIELD

The goal of yoga has always been to evolve *beyond* the body so
that we might tend to the higher priority of wrangling the mind
and, finally, elevating the spirit. We're encouraged to work hard and
challenge ourselves with the tricky asanas, but the real "trick" is to
be ourselves and to face life's challenges with compassion, humility,
and courage. We often sense this from the first time we are introduced to yoga—that the poses are part of something much greater—
yet finding what that something greater is for ourselves can be
challenging. This is precisely why yoga teachers are fond of saying,
"It's called a yoga *practice*, not a yoga perfect."

Today, there are as many reasons for doing yoga as there are people

who do it, every one as individual and personal as the shoes we leave
in a cubby outside the studio, worn and shaped by life, each pair
treading a unique path. The reasons we practice will not remain the
same. They evolve as we do. The difficulty for the modern yogi, then,
is learning to find ways to practice skills that are less visible but often more valuable. The growth of the yoga industry is admirable and
exciting, but what we see most often is not necessarily a reflection of
what we most need. Do I *need* to be able to touch my foot to my head in
King Pigeon to be happy? Do I need designer yoga clothes to experience inner peace? Certainly not. Do I need to wrangle my mind from
becoming too distracted, neurotic, or foreboding? Yes. Absolutely
yes. Yoga is a bit like the food industry that way. What we need most
is real food that nourishes us, but what we see more prominently are
foodlike products colorfully packaged and expertly marketed everywhere we turn. Yoga tasks us with using simple ingredients we were
all given at birth—our bodies, minds, and spirits—and combining
them in a way that fosters a nourishing life.

I'm not an anthropologist of any kind, nor an Indian philosophy
or yoga scholar, but yoga has nourished my life for a very long time.
(If my yoga years were a person, she'd be able to vote already—and
she would, since voting is the asana of democracy.) I lucked into being a precocious teenager who started doing yoga at the precise time
when its popularity in the United States started to explode, and I
paid close attention along the way. I organized this book to reflect
and support the journey of other modern yoga practitioners, who
eventually feel like they need more sustenance than what the average
asana class provides but aren't sure where to get it, can't quite relate
to traditional yoga philosophy in the midst of real life, or—let's face
it—they're not even sure what they need. What I almost forgot was
that one does yoga because one loves it.

I almost forgot that love itself is a spiritual practice and the ultimate form of sustenance. Love with a capital L, remember? It's spin-

ach to Popeye and cookies to Cookie Monster, and when done right, it makes us feel strong and joyful. That last part was something I had to learn while writing this book, during which time I both lost love and found it again, more potently than I've ever known. So, it stands to reason that love would literally be my final chapter. It has the last word. Love is the highest religion in the land and most acrobatic pose of them all—to launch your heart into the air, in the direction of someone or something else, in the direction of life itself—with no guarantee of what will happen next. It takes the yoga principles of letting go and having faith and puts them into practice, which is ideal since life is not lived theoretically or philosophically but practically.

I also learned something of love while attending a public meditation led by Thich Nhat Hanh, when he last visited Boston. I first came across the eighty-five-year-old Buddhist monk, peace activist, and author while taking an Eastern philosophy course in college. I still recall one of our homework assignments. We had to wash the dishes. My roommates were thrilled.

However, the assignment wasn't to wash the dishes the way any of us typically wash the dishes, dashing off a chore so that we can move on to something better, something interesting, something more worthwhile. Instead, the assignment required us to wash the dishes while being fully present and mindful. Forget about what happens next. We were learning through real-life practice that the powerful moment—the only one over which we have any guarantee or influence—is the one happening now. Don't wait until later to be loving or compassionate, attentive and aware. A mind does not get stronger that way. It stays distracted and anxious about what comes next . . . And after that . . . And then what?

Hundreds of people convened in Copley Square to hear Thich Nhat Hanh speak. It's the heart of Boston. Framing the perimeter of our gathering was the historic stone façade of Trinity Church; the John Hancock Tower, an iconic skyscraper; majestic statues and stairs that

lead to the Boston Public Library; and mere yards away, the Boston
Marathon finish line and vigil that formed and had expanded each
day since the bombing. Briefly, I wondered if what we were doing was
safe—so many of us congregated in an exposed area doing something
quasi-spiritual, so close to something so raw, geographically and
emotionally. I closed my eyes, feeling the sun on my face and letting
the moment's anxiety pass. It was a justified feeling but not helpful.
We waited for the beloved monk to speak. Many meditated. I heard
an airplane pass overhead. A few car horns honked in the distance. A
skateboarder cruised by.

The monk said nothing. He didn't even open his eyes. Instead,
he continued to sit silently in meditation for the next twenty-five
minutes, an unspoken signal for us to join him if we wanted. The
city seemed to join him, too. The traffic lulled. A few small children
giggled or cried briefly in the crowd, but mostly there was stillness.
I have to think that when you concentrate that many good intentions and focused minds in one place, there's a drafting effect, like
runners in a pack or cyclists in a peloton. Just as people can feed off
each other's energy and velocity, so, too, can we feed off collective
calmness.

When he eventually spoke, the famous monk began by saying only
this: *Breathing in, I am aware of my breath. Breathing out, I am aware of
my breath.* It was a simple mantra to set the stage for a talk that would
succinctly and poetically teach a diverse group what it means to be
mindful and how it creates peace. Next, he said: *Breathing in, I enjoy
breathing in. Breathing out, I enjoy breathing out.*

The mantras and teachings gained momentum from there. We
breathed in and out qualities of a mountain's solidity and stability,
water's stillness and reflection, a flower's freshness and beauty, and
space. *Breathing in, I have the element of space within me. Breathing out,
I feel free . . . Space: free.* I was reminded of each of the chakras and
koshas, the way yoga believes that the body, too, is made up of all the

elements of the earth, and our job is to balance them, as well as integrate all its layers. Yet, nothing was too heady and no one was left out of this special talk. It was the simplest yet most moving talk I've ever witnessed on meditation.

Then, the talk moved into the territory of love, which I may not have predicted from an elderly celibate monk. It could have easily represented love for a family member or friend, but to hear a monk use the word *darling* in three different types of mantras suggested something of romantic love, and it made everyone smile. *Darling, I am here. Darling, I know you are here. Darling, I know that you suffer, and I am here for you.* He continued, "The most precious thing you can offer your loved one is your presence. To be present means to be there. How can you love, if you are not there?" His voice was gentle, but the message reverberated. Love (romantic or otherwise) doesn't work if we're distracted or hiding—behind suffering, the screen of a computer or phone, the fuzziness of alcohol, the busyness of work. We all have our means of avoiding pain and seeking pleasure, some healthier than others. To love means to understand suffering, our own and our darling's, and to truly show up in a given moment. Yoga, it can be said, helps us fully show up.

Finally, Thich Nhat Hanh linked the two segments of the talk seamlessly: the meditation, breathing, and mantras with his thoughts on love. We practice meditation so that we can restore our presence and feel more stable, free, fresh, and beautiful, he told us. "You cannot buy it in a market"—the adorable monk cautioned in his lilting accent—the level of presence required for true love. "You have to produce it yourself." The same can be said for true anything. Happiness. Peace. Even beauty. They're all products of the deeper business of being in full possession of who and what we are.

Spiritual pursuits, like yoga and meditation, sometimes receive criticism for being selfish or self-indulgent when the opposite is actually true. If we are healthy in body, clear in mind, and in touch with our spirits, we can be all those things for others. We are fortified. We know that life will be hard, and, yet, we have a reservoir of strength to share with the world. Each relationship we have—personal, professional, familial, communal, or romantic—can be a vehicle for respect and connection. More than anything, this is what we seek—to be happy and to feel like we belong. Deep down, we know that the purpose of yoga isn't to become really good at yoga, it's to make our lives better by being more connected, to ourselves, each other, and the moment. Only then, can we truly fall in love with any of them.

The End and the Beginning

This is where *Do Your Om Thing* comes to an end, and doing *your* om thing continues. It will take many forms, and it is whatever you make it. Some days the yoga path is full of love and light, bliss and abundance. Other days it's mundane or even miserable. Funny thing about yoga being part of real life, isn't it? Some days your body is injured, or maybe it's your spirit. The rent is due. The kids are sick, or the unfathomable happens. The dreaded phone call comes, one that makes you wince at how easy life was before.

But, if you can breathe, you can do yoga, on your mat or anywhere else. You can connect—to yourself, the environment, the present moment, and others. Yoga won't alter reality, which is challenging for everyone at some point, even those who can stand on their hands, meditate daily, or chug kale juice. Yoga influences how we see and *respond* to reality. It shows us what we're made of—physically, energetically, emotionally, intellectually, and spiritually—and can remake a person in the image of stronger stuff. *It stills the fluctuations of the mind.*

Using yoga, you can shift your attitude about the world and yourself. You can delight in the paradox of using the body to figure out that you are not your body. You can stretch your mind and befriend yourself in any given moment. You can "wake up" like a buddha. You can look at life as a complex asana you never thought you'd be able to do but now accomplish effortlessly. Size it up. Break it down. See it clearly. Then, practice. Practice putting it all together, using this ancient system of health care for body, mind, and spirit. Synthesize your yoga experience with your real-life wisdom, and you will find a fresh form of success—the enlightened state of knowing that it's a privilege to be you. It's a victory we forget we always have on lock: there's no one more *youer than you.*

So, what will your om thing be? Is it just asanas on a mat? Or, is it something bigger, bolder, and evolving? Does it feel more portable, fluid, and connected now? This is my hope. Life is stressful, and it would be a shame if the only way you could reap the benefits of yoga was by attending a class. What if you're on a bumpy airplane or in a contentious work meeting? What if your schedule simply doesn't jive with that of a yoga studio? What if you have a baby who doesn't abide by a yoga-studio schedule, either? Unrolling your mat in the work meeting as tempers flare isn't an option. The baby doesn't care that your favorite teacher is on the schedule tonight.

Take heart, modern yogis. You can breathe deeply on the bumpy airplane. You might recite mantras while lulling the fussy baby. You should feel free to love and participate in other forms of fitness. Yoga doesn't have to be your sole workout. It can be your soul work-out. This is your path. You get to decide. You respect the yogis who've walked before you—their culture, wisdom, intentions, and commitment. You honor the light in every teacher and other yogi you meet. You try, at least. You bow to the Divine in everyone whenever you can, but you also don't have to like everyone. Find a way to make *life* the practice—one of humility, gratitude, and awareness. And the next time someone says that yoga means more than the poses, you won't just agree, pleasantly and theoretically. You will know it in the core of your being, which flickers with the spark of all other beings, that this is true. You'll know why and how to practice this truth, rather than merely saying it. This is what we mean when we chant *om*. It's a nod to what binds and brightens us, individually and as part of a collective. It's the vibration of the whole universe as one, in which each of us occupy a small corner, where we do our best, live our fullest, and do our om thing.

Acknowledgments

First, I bow deeply to the tradition of yoga, ancient and evolving, and to all my teachers, past and present, of yoga (on the mat and off), meditation, and writing; especially those who appear in these pages, including but not limited to (chronologically) Carol Dubin, Valerie Jeremijenko, Dr. Miranda Shaw, Baron Baptiste, Patricia Walden, Deepak Chopra, and Jon Kabat-Zinn. I am indebted to and humbled by my students, readers of omgal.com, members of OG Book Club, and the yoga community around the world and in my home of Boston. You inspire me endlessly. To the institutions that fostered my lifelong love of books and desire to be a writer, of which the Loomis Chaffee School and University of Richmond are chief among them, I treasure your guidance always.

Thank you to my literary agents, Kathryn Beaumont Murphy and Katherine Flynn and the impeccable team at Kneerim, Williams & Bloom. You made this life dream come true and supported me every step of the way. Kathryn, your heart and mind are the mightiest of combinations, and from our first meeting, I was honored to have them in my corner. Katherine, you helped me stay the course when my doubts attempted to get the best of me. I feel so lucky to have landed in your care. To the primary reader and personal champion of this manuscript, Priscilla Warner, I am forever grateful. I, too, am happy neither of us is ageist because you are the most fabulous sixtysomething author friend a thirtysomething gal could have. You sparked a new appreciation for radishes, implored me to trust my voice, and taught me, with great aplomb, to say *eff it* on occasion. To my editor, Julie Will, you were my guru from start to finish. Thank you for the precision, direction, and confidence you lent me along the way. It was an honor and privilege to work with you. Karen Rinaldi, you are a force. Thank you for making me one of your authors. Sydney Pierce, Liz Esman, Katie O'Callaghan, Leah Carlson-Stanisic, Milan Bozic, and everyone else at HarperWave, thank you for supporting me, bringing our vision to life, and making it possible for me to do *my* om thing. Jonathan Pozniak, my longtime friend and talented photographer, I am so happy our karma continues to intersect. I hope it does for many lifetimes of mischief and making art. Thank you for your beautiful studio in which to shoot in NYC, James Weber. Matt Osbourne (my ambassador of hip), Christine Needham, Daren Bascome, and my friends at Proverb, just being in your company fed my creative fire. Thank you for your design input. To the partnerships that have supported me and helped grow my business, namely Equinox, Inner Strength, lululemon, and *Runner's World,* I am deeply grateful. Finally, thank you to my smart and soulful Om Experts, Derek Beres, Mallika Chopra, and Kim Vandenberg, for your thoughtful contributions to this book. It is better, and the world is a brighter, more informed and inspired place because of you.

To my family. Thank you for your love and support. Mom and Dad, you always encouraged me to leave things better than I found them, so I'm giving it a try with my small corner of the universe. I hope this book makes yoga and life a little better or easier for those who read it. Gram, thank you for your unconditional love and passing down a love for the spiritual realm. Reece, you are one of my life's great gifts—a brother I would have chosen but didn't need to.

To my friends. You were with me in spirit on every page. I love you with all my heart. Thank you, in particular, to those who sheltered me (emotionally and literally) while I was working on my manuscript, Abigail Erdmann and Luc Aalmans. Serena Kabat-Zinn and Coeli Marsh, thank you for sharing your feedback, wit, wisdom, and the uplifting company of your beautiful children. You have been bright lights (torches, really) on my yoga journey for a long time. Emma Barton, Chanel Luck, and Larisa Forman, extraordinary yogis, I trust you implicitly and thank you deeply. Cynthia Pham Gordon, you were the first to read page one and cheered this labor of love for years. Vinita Goswami, I will always cherish our board meetings.

To Dan. I started writing this book long before we met, but you are the one who truly taught me to live it. You make my heart feel whole and brave. My next chapter will always start with you. I love you.

Glossary

Abyasa: practice, discipline.

Ahimsa: non-violence, non-harming, the first yama.

Aparigaha: greedlessness, the fifth yama.

Asana: used interchangeably as the word for a yoga pose or posture, literally means *seat*.

Ashram: place of retreat devoted to the spiritual path of yoga.

Ashtanga: refers to the eight-limbed path (ashta = eight, anga = limb), proposed by Patanjali. As a proper noun, it refers to a precise and vigorous style of yoga created by the late Pattabhi Jois, the precursor to popular offshoots such as Vinyasa and Power Yoga.

Asteya: non-stealing, the third yama.

Atman: self or soul.

Bhagavad Gita: 700-verse epic included in the *Mahabharata*, featuring the story of Arjuna going to battle.

Bhakti: devotion.

Brahmacharya: celibacy, abstinence, the fourth yama.

Chakra: wheel of light, most commonly referring to seven major psychoenergetic centers along the spine, which conduct energy along the body's central axis or spine.

Dharana: concentration, the sixth of the eight limbs.

Dharma: sacred duty or calling.

Dhyana: meditation, the seventh of the eight limbs and precursor to enlightenment (samadhi).

Drishti: gaze.

Ishvara Pranidhana: surrender to God, the practice of having faith, and fifth niyama.

Iyengar: refers to a style of yoga created by B.K.S. Iyengar, a key figure in the proliferation and popularity of modern yoga. This style of practice is known for being meticulous, alignment focused, and favoring the use of props.

Japa: meditation style using mantras.

Karma: action.

Kosha: sheath or layer of the subtle body; there are five sheaths.

Maha: great, supreme.

Mahabharata: One of two national epics of India (the other is the *Ramayana*), featuring some of the earliest mentions of yoga. Scholars debate the exact date of its origin. Georg Feuerstein surmises that the date was around 200 CE.

Mantra: syllable, word, or phrase used to anchor the mind in meditation, of which om is the most popular. Mantra literally means "mind protecting," as in a conscious thought we give the mind to help it focus rather than get lost in distraction or reactivity.

Metta: loving-kindness, unconditional love.

Mudra: seal, as in sealing in an intention, most often using the hands in a specific gesture of meaning and focus.

Niyamas: attitudes toward the self, the second of the eight limbs.

Om: sacred syllable said to contain the sound of the whole universe. It represents connection, oneness, and the Divine.

Padma: lotus, symbolic in Eastern traditions as a beautiful flower grown from muddy waters.

Prana: breath, life force.

Pranayama: breathwork, the fourth of the eight limbs.

Pratyhara: withdrawal of the senses, the fifth of the eight limbs.

Puja: worship, commonly referring to a morning/daily ritual of sitting in prayer or meditation before a self-made altar of sacred objects, candles, to name two popular choices.

Ramayana: One of two national epics of India (the other is the *Mahabharata*), featuring the tale of Rama.

Samadhi: the final limb of the yoga path, known commonly as enlightenment, ecstasy, or superconsciousness. It means, "to stand inside of" as in one's true Self.

Sangha: spiritual community of friends and sages.

Santosha: contentment, the second niyama.

Satya: truthfulness, the second yama.

Saucha: purity, cleanliness, the first niyama.

Shanti: peace.

Sutra: thread. Most notably as in *The Yoga Sutras of Patanjali*, a foundational yogic text.

Svadhyaya: self-study, the fourth niyama.

Tapas: heat, purifying fire, or glow, the third niyama.

Tratak: the act of staring at an object in meditation to cleanse the eyes.

Upanishads: genre of Hindu literature dating back before Common Era.

Vairagya: letting go.

Vinyasa: to flow. When used as a proper noun, refers to the style of yoga most popular in the United States at the time of publication.

Yamas: attitudes toward the world, the first of the eight limbs.

Recommended Resources

Asana

Baptiste, Baron. *Journey into Power*. New York: Simon & Schuster, 2002.

Birch, Beryl Bender. *Power Yoga*. New York: Simon & Schuster, 1995.

Hirschi, Gertrud. *Mudras: Yoga in Your Hands*. York Beach, ME: Red Wheel Weiser, 2000.

Iyengar, B.K.S. *Light on Yoga*. New York: Random House, 1966.

Iyengar, B.K.S. *Yoga: The Path to Holistic Health*. London: Dorling Kindersley, 2001.

The Body

Judith, Anodea. *Eastern Body, Western Mind*. New York: Crown, 1996.

Kaminoff, Leslie. *Yoga Anatomy*. Champaign, IL: Human Kinetics, 2007.

Lad, Vasant. *The Complete Book of Ayurvedic Home Remedies*. New York: Crown, 1998.

Meditation

Hanh, Thich Nhat. *Miracle of Mindfulness*. Boston: Beacon Press, 1975.

Kabat-Zinn, Jon. *Wherever You Go There You Are*. New York: Hyperion, 1994.

Mental Health

Chodron, Pema. *When Things Fall Apart*. Boston: Shambhala, 2005.

Forbes, Bo. *Yoga for Emotional Balance*. Boston: Shambhala, 2011.

Nutrition

Telpner, Meghan. *Undiet*. Guilford, CT: Globe Pequot Press, 2013.

Philosophy and Tradition

Easwaran, Eknath. *The Upanishads*. Tomales, CA: Nilgiri Press, 1987.

Feuerstein, Georg. *The Shambhala Encyclopedia of Yoga*. Boston: Shambhala, 1997.

Lasater, Judith. *Living Your Yoga*. Berkeley, CA: Rodmell Press, 2000.

Satchidananda, Sri Swami. *The Yoga Sutras of Patanjali*. Yogaville, VA: Integral Yoga Publications, 1978.

Stoler Miller, Barbara. *The Bhagavad Gita*. New York: Bantam, 1986.

Spirituality

Chopra, Deepak. *7 Spiritual Laws of Success*. Novato, CA: New World Library, 1994.

Lamott, Anne. *Help, Thanks, Wow: The Three Essential Prayers*. New York: Riverhead Books, 2012.

Moore, Thomas. *Care of the Soul*. New York: HarperCollins, 1992.

Myss, Caroline. *Anatomy of the Spirit*. New York: Crown, 1996.

Visualization

Gawain, Shakti. *Creative Visualization*. Novato, CA: New World Library, 1978.

Bibliography

Arnold, Carrie. "Gut Feelings: The Future of Psychiatry May be in Your Stomach." *The Verge*, August 2013.

Baptiste, Baron. *Journey into Power*. New York: Simon & Schuster, 2002.

Barcott, Bruce. "Mind Gains." *Runner's World*. February 2010.

"Blue Light has a Dark Side." *Harvard Health Publications*. May 2012.

Bormann, J.E., T.L. Smith, S. Becker, M. Gershwin, L. Pada, A. Grudzinski, et al. (2005). "Efficacy of frequent mantram repetition on stress, quality of life, and spiritual well-being in veterans: A pilot study." *Journal of Holistic Nursing*, 23(4), 394-413.

Brown, Brené. *Daring Greatly*. New York: Gotham, 2012.

Brown, R.P., P.L. Gerbag. "Yoga Breathing, Meditation, and Longevity." *Annals of the New York Academy of Sciences*. 2009, 1172:54-62.

Campbell, Joseph. *The Hero with a Thousand Faces*. New York: Pantheon, 1949.

Cuddy, Amy. "Your Body Language Shapes Who Your Are." TED.com, October 2012.

Devananda, Swami Vishnu. *The Complete Illustrated Book of Yoga*. New York: Crown, 1960.

Driver, Janine. *You Say More Than You Think*. New York: Crown, 2010.

Easwaran, Eknath. *The Upanishads*. Tomales, CA: Nilgiri Press, 1987.

Feuerstein, Georg. *The Shambhala Encyclopedia of Yoga*. Boston: Shambhala, 1997.

Forbes, Bo. *Yoga for Emotional Balance*. Boston: Shambhala, 2011.

Gladwell, Malcolm. *Blink*. New York: Little Brown, 2005.

Hölzel, K. Britta, James Carmody, Mark Vangel, Christina Congleton, Sita M. Yerramsetti, Tim Gard, Sara W. Lazar. "Mindfulness Practice Leads to Increases in Regional Brain Gray Matter Density." *Psychiatry Research: Neuroimaging*, 2011; 191 (1): 36 DOI: 10.1016/j.pscychresns.2010.08.006.

Kabat-Zinn, Jon. *Wherever You Go There You Are*. New York: Hyperion, 1994.

Kornfield, Jack. *After the Ecstasy, The Laundry*. New York: Bantam, 2000.

Lasater, Judith. *Living Your Yoga*. Berkeley, CA: Rodmell Press, 2000.

Rubin, Gretchen. *The Happiness Project*. New York: HarperCollins, 2009.

Satchidananada, Sri Swami. T*he Yoga Sutras of Patanjali*. Yogaville, VA: Integral Yoga Publications, 1978.

Stoler Miller, Barbara. *The Bhagavad Gita*. New York: Bantam, 1986.

Telpner, Meghan. *Undiet*. Guilford, CT: Globe Pequot Press, 2013.

Vienne, Veronique, Erica Lennard. *The Art of Doing Nothing*. New York: Crown, 1998.

About the Author

Rebecca Pacheco is an acclaimed yoga teacher, writer, speaker, and creator of the popular yoga blog OmGal.com. She has been practicing yoga for more than half her lifetime and began teaching while studying English literature at the University of Richmond. Previously a master teacher at the Baptiste Power Yoga Institute, Rebecca now blends nearly two decades of yoga experience into her signature Om Athlete and creative Vinyasa classes. A longtime runner and Boston Marathon finisher, she is also the resident yoga expert for *Runner's World* magazine's online Yoga Center.

In addition to teaching internationally, Rebecca has had the honor of leading the first-ever yoga class on the field at Fenway Park. She lives in Boston with her fiancé, Dan Fitzgerald.

You can connect with Rebecca on social media @omgal.